Student Study Guide

to accompany

Kinn's **The Administrative Medical Assistant**

An Applied Learning Approach

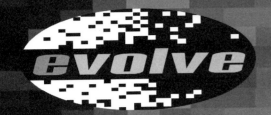

The Latest *Evolution* in Learning.

Evolve provides online access to free learning resources and activities designed specifically for the textbook you are using in your class. The resources will provide you with information that enhances the material covered in the book and much more.

Visit the Web address listed below to start your learning evolution today!

▶ **LOGIN:** *http://evolve.elsevier.com/Kinn/*

Evolve Student Learning Resources for Morton: Student Study Guide to accompany Kinn's The Administrative Medical Assistant: An Applied Learning Approach, *5th Edition* offer the following features:

- **Content Updates**
  The latest content updates from the authors of the textbook to keep you current with recent developments in medical assisting, updated procedures, and more!

- **Online Quizzes**
  Quizzes for each chapter are set up for instant feedback, any time you want a little practice.

- **Weblinks**
  An exciting resource that lets you link to hundreds of websites carefully chosen to supplement the content of the textbook and student study guide. The Weblinks are regularly updated, with new ones added as they develop.

- **Chapter Resources**
  Additional materials, including chapter summaries and suggested readings, to enhance each chapter.

- **Study Tips**
  Get advice on how to maximize study time and review material for optimal results. Discover your individual learning style and find out how it applies to your ability to learn new material.

Think outside the book... *evolve*

Student Study Guide

to accompany

Kinn's **The Administrative Medical Assistant**

An Applied Learning Approach

FIFTH EDITION

Tammy B. Morton, MS, RN, CS, CMA

Formerly Department Head, Medical Assisting Program
TriCounty Technical College
Pendleton, South Carolina

SAUNDERS
An Imprint of Elsevier Science

SAUNDERS
An Imprint of Elsevier Science
11830 Westline Industrial Drive
St. Louis, Missouri 63146

Student Study Guide to Accompany
Kinn's The Administrative Medical Assistant: An Applied Learning Approach, 5th edition   0-7216-0052-2

This Study Guide is dedicated to
my family, friends, and former students
who have encouraged and supported me
throughout my teaching career.

Many thanks to Karen Sorrow, Kathy Duncan, Mary Heyer, Adrianne Cochran, Christine Ambrose, and Jeanne Genz for helping make the project a success.

Executive Editor: Adrianne Cochran
Developmental Editor: Christine Ambrose
Publishing Services Manager: Gayle May
Designer: Mark Oberkrom

Printed in the United States of America

CE/MV-B

Last digit is print number: 9   8   7   6   5   4   3   2   1

To the Student

This study guide was created to assist you in achieving the objectives of each chapter in *The Administrative Medical Assistant: An Applied Learning Approach* and in establishing a solid base of knowledge in medical assisting. Completing the exercises in each chapter in this guide will help to reinforce the material studied in the textbook and learned in class.

Study Hints for All Students

Ask Questions!

There are no stupid questions. If you do not know something or are not sure about it, you need to find out. Other people may be wondering the same thing but may be too shy to ask. The answer could mean life or death to your patient. That is certainly more important than feeling embarrassed about asking a question.

Chapter Objectives

At the beginning of each chapter in the textbook are learning objectives that you should have mastered when you finish studying that chapter. Write these objectives in your notebook, leaving a blank space after each. Fill in the answers as you find them while reading the chapter. Review to make sure your answers are correct and complete. Use these answers when you study for tests. This should also be done for separate course objectives that your instructor has listed in your class syllabus.

Vocabulary

At the beginning of each chapter in the textbook are vocabulary terms that you will encounter as you read the chapter. These vocabulary terms are in bold the first time they appear in the chapter.

Summary of Learning Objectives

Use the Summary of Learning Objectives at the end of each chapter in the textbook to help with review for exams.

Reading Hints

When reading each chapter in the textbook, look at the subject headings to learn what each section is about. Read first for the general meaning. Then reread parts you did not understand. It may help to read those parts aloud. Carefully read the information given in each table and study each figure and its legend.

Concepts

While studying, put difficult concepts into your own words to determine whether you understand them. Check this understanding with another student or the instructor. Write these concepts in your notebook.

Class Notes

When taking lecture notes in class, leave a large margin on the left side of each notebook page and write only on right-hand pages, leaving all left-hand pages blank. Look over your lecture notes soon after each class, while your memory is fresh. Fill in missing words; complete sentences and ideas; and underline key phrases, definitions, and concepts. At the top of each page, write the topic of that page. In the left margin, write the key word for that part of your notes. On the opposite left-hand page, write a summary or outline that combines material from both the textbook and the lecture. These can be your study notes for review.

Study Groups

Form a study group with some other students so you can help one another. Practice speaking and reading aloud. Ask questions about material you are not sure about. Work together to find answers.

References for Improving Study Skills

Good study skills are essential for achieving your goals in medical assisting. Time management, efficient use of study time, and a consistent approach to studying are all beneficial. There are various methods for reading a textbook and for taking class notes. Some methods that have proven helpful can be found in *Saunders Health Professional's Planner*.

Additional Study Hints for English as a Second Language (ESL) Students

Vocabulary

If you find a nontechnical word you do not know (e.g., drowsy), try to guess its meaning from the sentence (e.g., *With electrolyte imbalance, the patient may feel fatigued and drowsy*). If you are not sure of the meaning or if it seems particularly important, look it up in the dictionary.

Vocabulary Notebook

Keep a small alphabetized notebook or address book in your pocket or purse. Write down new nontechnical words you read or hear along with their meanings and pronunciations. Write each word under its initial letter so you can find it easily, as in a dictionary. For words you do not know or for words that have a different meaning in medical assisting, write down how they are used and how they sound. Look up their meanings in a dictionary or ask your instructor or first-language buddy. Then write the different meanings or usages that you have found in your book, including the medical assisting meaning. Continue to add new words as you discover them.

First-Language Buddy

ESL students should find a first-language buddy—another student who is a native speaker of English and who is willing to answer questions about word meanings, pronunciations, and culture. Maybe, in turn, your buddy would like to learn about your language and culture. This could be useful for his or her medical assisting experience as well.

Introduction

This student study guide is designed with Learning Style Icons to help you identify exercises that will appeal to your strengths and weaknesses. Over time you have developed a method for perceiving and processing information. This pattern of behavior is called your learning style. There are many different ways of examining learning styles but professionals agree that success of students has more to do with their ability to "make sense" of the information rather than whether or not they are "smart". Education that is based on attention to individual learning styles is sensitive to the different ways students learn and approach new material with a wide variety of methods so that all students have the opportunity to learn. Determining your individual learning style and understanding how it applies to your ability to learn new material is the first step to becoming a successful student.

To learn new material, two things have to happen. First is your perception of the information. This is the method you have developed over time that helps you examine the material and recognize it as real. The next step is to process the information. Processing the information is how you internalize it and make it your own. Investigating various learning styles tells you how you can combine different methods of perceiving and processing information. In his book *Becoming a Master Student*, David Ellis discusses these different methods of information perception, processing, and learning.*

Information perception involves how you go about examining new material and making it real. There are two ways learners perceive new material. Some people are concrete perceivers who learn information through direct experience by doing, acting, sensing, or feeling. Concrete learners prefer to learn things that have a personal meaning or things they feel are relevant and important to them. Other learners are abstract perceivers who take in information through analysis, observation, and reflection. Abstract learners like to think things through. They analyze the new material and build theories to help understand it. They prefer structured learning situations and use a step-by-step approach to problem solving.

Information processing is how you internalize the new information and make it your own. There are also two different methods for processing material. Active processors prefer to jump in and start doing things immediately. They make sense of the new material by immediately using it. They look for practical ways to apply the new material and typically don't mind taking risks to get the desired results. They learn best with practice and hands-on activities. Reflective processors, however, have to think about the information before they can internalize it. They prefer to observe and consider what is going on. The only way they can make sense of new material is to spend time thinking about it and learning a great deal of information about it before acting.

*Ellis D: Becoming a master student, ed 10, Boston, 2002, Houghton Mifflin.

None of us fall completely into one or the other of these categories. However, by being aware of how we generally prefer to first perceive information and then process it, we can be more sensitive to our learning style and approach new learning situations with a plan for learning the material in a way that best suits our learning preferences. Your preferred perceiving/processing learning profile will fall into one of the following stages.

Learners in Stage 1 have a concrete/reflective style. and These students want to know the purpose of the information and have a personal connection to the content. They like to consider a situation from many different points of view, observe others, and plan before taking action. Their strengths are in understanding people, brainstorming, and recognizing and creatively solving problems. If you fall into this stage you enjoy small group activities and learn well in study groups.

Stage 2 learners have an abstract/reflective style. and These students are eager to learn just for the sheer pleasure of learning rather than because the material relates to their personal lives. They like to learn lots of facts and arrange new material in a logical and clear manner. Stage 2 learners plan studying and like to create ways of thinking about the material but don't always make the connection with the practical application of the material. If you are a Stage 2 learner you prefer organized, logical presentations of material and, therefore, enjoy lectures and generally dislike group work. You also need time to process and think about the new material before applying it.

Learners in Stage 3 have an abstract/active style. and Learners with this combination of learning style want to experiment and test the knowledge they are learning. If you are a Stage 3 learner you want to know how techniques or ideas work buy you also want to practice what you are learning. Your strengths are in problem solving and making decisions but you may tend to lack focus and be hasty in your decision-making. You learn best with hands-on practice by doing experiments, projects, and lab activities. You also enjoy working alone or in small groups.

Stage 4 is made up of concrete/active learners. and Students in this stage are concerned about how they can use what they learn to make a difference in their lives. If you fall into this stage, you like to relate new material to other areas of your life. You have leadership capabilities, can create on your feet, and are usually vocal in a group but you may have difficulty getting your work done completely and on time. Stage 4 learners enjoy teaching others and working in groups and learn best when they can apply the new information to real-world problems.

To get the most out of knowing your learning profile you need to apply this knowledge to how you approach learning. There are plusses and minuses to all four of the learning stages. When faced with a learning situation that does not match your learning preference, see how you can adapt your individual learning to make the best of the information. For example, if you are bored by lectures, look for an opportunity to apply the information being presented into a real-world problem you are facing in the classroom or at home. When learning new material, if you are an abstract perceiver, take time outside of class to think about the information, so you are ready to process it into your learning system. If you benefit from learning in a group, then make the effort to organize review sessions and study groups with other interested students. If you learn best by teaching others offer to assist your peers with their learning. Take time now to investigate your preferred method of learning and it will help you perceive and process information more effectively throughout your school career.

Contents

Procedure Checklists

CHAPTER 1

Becoming a Successful Student

Part I. Vocabulary

A. **Directions:** Match the following terms and definitions.

1. _____ The constant practice of considering all aspects of a situation when deciding what to believe or what to do.

2. _____ Those actions that identify the medical assistant as a member of a healthcare profession, including dependability, respectful patient care, initiative, positive attitude, and teamwork.

3. _____ How an individual looks at information and sees it as real.

4. _____ The way that an individual perceives and processes information to learn new material.

5. _____ How an individual internalizes new information and makes it his or her own.

6. _____ The process of considering new information and internalizing it to create new ways of examining information.

7. _____ Sensitivity to the individual needs and reactions of patients.

A. learning style

B. reflection

C. professional behaviors

D. processing

E. empathy

F. perceiving

G. critical thinking

B. **Directions:** Complete the following sentences by using the vocabulary words from the previous section correctly.

1. Jo uses _____ _____ when she decides which information to use when she instructs patients with newly diagnosed diabetes.

2. _____ _____ should always be displayed during the student externship experience.

3. Instructors attempt to design lessons that appeal to different _____

   _____.

4. Amanda shows _____ when she expresses concern about a patient's illness.

5. Sam enjoys "hands-on" learning activities. He uses an active style of _____ information.

6. Concrete and abstract are two ways of _____ new information.

Part II. Learning Style Inventory

Directions: Using the descriptions of various learning styles from Chapter 1, insert the correct Learning Style Stage Number into the diagram below by correlating the processing and perceiving style. In his book, *Becoming a Master Student,* Ellis discusses these different methods of information perception, processing, and learning.*

	Processing	
	Watching (Reflective)	Doing (Active)
Perceiving		
Feeling (Concrete)	Stage _____	Stage _____
Thinking (Abstract)	Stage _____	Stage _____

Part III. Time Management

1. List five time management skills.

    a. _____

    b. _____

    c. _____

    d. _____

    e. _____

2. Describe five strategies for breaking the cycle of procrastination.

    a. _____

    b. _____

    c. _____

    d. _____

    e. _____

*Ellis D: Becoming a master student, ed 10, Boston, 2002, Houghton Mifflin.

Part IV. Conflict Resolution

Directions: Indicate which statements are true (T) and which statements are false (F).

1. _____ The best way to deal with conflict situations is through open, honest, assertive communication.

2. _____ The first step in conflict resolution is examination of pros and cons.

3. _____ Conflicts should be resolved immediately.

4. _____ Sometimes you will not be able to solve problems or a conflict may not be important enough for you to act to change it.

5. _____ It is best if you attempt to solve the conflict in a private place at a prescheduled time.

6. _____ You need to understand the problem and gather as much information about the situation as possible before you decide to act.

7. _____ As a future member of the healthcare team, you will frequently face problems and conflict.

Part V. Workplace Applications

Scenario: Connie is the manager of a busy family practice office. The insurance clerk has complained that the receptionist takes too many smoking breaks and accepts too many personal calls while at work.

Step One: Think about this situation and how you believe it should be handled. Record your ideas.

_____

_____

_____

_____

Step Two: Pair up with a classmate and discuss your ideas. Record ideas on which you agree and compare them with those in the text.

_____

_____

_____

_____

_____

Step Three: Share your ideas with your classmates. Make notes of any ideas that you did not think of before.

_____

_____

_____

_____

_____

Part VI. Study Skills

Examine your own note-taking ability. Review the note-taking strategies in Chapter 1, and record the ideas that you plan to incorporate into your academic goals for this term.

_____

_____

_____

_____

_____

_____

_____

_____

Directions: Complete the following success checklist.

	Yes	No
1. I am prepared for class.		
2. My notebook is organized.		
3. I read my assignments before coming to class.		
4. I attend all classes.		
5. I listen most of the time.		
6. I arrive early to class.		
7. I date notes in my notebook.		
8. I save all papers and course materials for review.		
9. I try to connect what I read in the text with what I learn in class.		
10. My schoolwork is a high priority.		

If you answered "No" to any of the items on the checklist, write a short plan for improvement in this area.

_____

_____

_____

_____

_____

Part VII. Test-Taking Strategies

Directions: Complete the following sentences.

1. The first step of taking charge of your academic success is to

_____

_____.

2. Before you begin a test _____.

Chapter 1 Quiz

Name: _____

1. List three examples of professional behaviors.

   a. _____

   b. _____

   c. _____

2. _____ is showing sensitivity to the individual needs and reactions of patients.

3. The process of considering new information and internalizing it to create new ways of examining information is called

   _____.

4. Initial confrontations regarding conflicts in the office should be done in

   _____.

5. True or False: Concrete learners enjoy theories and facts.

6. True or False: Active learning involves "hands-on" experiences.

7. List Two ways to use effective time management.

   a. _____

   b. _____

8. Give an example of a mind map.

   _____

CHAPTER 2

The Healthcare Industry

Part I. The History Of Medicine

Directions: Fill in the blanks. Use the Word Find below for clues.

1. The mythological staff belonging to Apollo, the _____, which is a staff encircled by two serpents, is the medical insignia of the United States Army Medical Corps and is often misused as a symbol of the medical profession.

2. _____ presented rules of health to the Jews around 1205 BC. He was thus the first advocate of preventive medicine and is considered the first public health officer.

3. _____, known as the father of medicine, is the most famous of the ancient Greek physicians. He is best remembered for an oath that has been taken by many physicians for more than 2000 years.

4. _____ was a Greek physician who migrated to Rome in 162 AD and became known as the prince of physicians.

5. _____ was a Belgian anatomist who is known as the father of modern anatomy.

6. In 1628, _____ announced his discovery that the heart acts as a muscular pump, forcing and propelling the blood throughout the body.

7. _____ was the first to observe bacteria and protozoa through a lens.

8. The famous English scientist, _____, is known as the founder of scientific surgery.

9. _____ observed that those who had contracted cowpox never contracted smallpox.

10. _____ directed that in his wards, the students were to wash and disinfect their hands before going to examine women in labor and deliver infants.

11. _____ saved the dairy industry of France during the nineteenth century from disaster by a process now called *pasteurization*, immortalizing his name.

12. _____ reasoned that microorganisms must be the cause of infection and should be kept out of wounds.

13. _____ was the first to use ether as an anesthetic agent.

14. Marie and Pierre _____ discovered radium in 1898, and they were awarded the 1902 Nobel Prize in Physics for their work on radioactivity.

15. _____ is known as the founder of nursing and fondly called "the lady with the lamp."

16. In 1881, _____ organized a committee in Washington, forming the American Red Cross.

17. _____ became the American leader of the birth control movement.

18. _____ wrote about death and dying.

19. Salk and _____ almost eradicated polio, which was once the killer and crippler of thousands in the United States.

20. David _____, MD, is considered by many to be one of the most brilliant minds today; he has helped to piece together the puzzle of the human immunodeficiency virus (HIV).

21. During his terms as the Surgeon General of the United States, _____ became a proponent of tobacco awareness, insisting that tobacco advertisements must be made less attractive to the youth of today.

Word Find

Directions: Use your answers above and find the names.

S	K	H	U	N	T	E	R	Q	T	W	L
E	E	O	S	S	O	R	E	N	N	E	J
M	O	L	O	H	M	E	I	B	C	V	M
M	H	I	P	P	O	C	R	A	T	E	S
E	N	S	C	Y	S	A	U	R	C	S	A
L	E	T	K	E	E	D	C	T	E	A	N
W	W	E	H	V	S	U	K	O	G	L	G
E	U	R	I	R	T	C	V	N	X	I	E
I	E	J	G	A	L	E	N	O	Z	U	R
S	E	E	K	H	W	U	P	B	X	S	K
S	L	O	N	G	V	S	A	B	I	N	M
E	L	A	G	N	I	T	H	G	I	N	Y

Part II. Acronyms in Health Care

Directions: Spell out the following acronyms.

1. WHO _____ _____ _____

2. DHHS _____ _____ and _____ _____

3. USAMRIID _____ _____ _____ _____

    _____ of _____ _____

4. CDC _____ for _____ _____ and

    _____

5. NIH _____ _____ of _____

6. CLIA _____ _____ _____ _____

7. OSHA _____ _____ and _____ _____

Part III. Practices and Practitioners

Directions: Use the appropriate terms to complete the sentences.

1. Dr. Hazlehurst has responsibility for her practice seven days a week. This practice is called a

   _____ _____.

2. A _____ is when two or more physicians elect to associate in the practice of medicine; they may enter into a partnership agreement.

3. Dr. Sorrow and Dr. Wester sold their practice, and now they work for a _____.

4. A _____ is trained to locate subluxations of the spine and repair them, using x-ray examinations and adjustments.

5. _____ physicians, or DOs, complete requirements similar to those for medical doctors to graduate and practice medicine.

6. Duncan wants to become a _____ that treats and prevents problems dealing with the teeth, gums, and tissue surrounding them.

7. You need new eyeglasses. You call an _____ because he or she is trained and licensed to examine the eyes to test visual acuity and to treat defects of vision by prescribing correctional lenses and other optical aids.

8. Your physician-employer has asked you to set up an appointment with a _____ because he or she is educated in caring for the feet, including surgical treatment.

9. _____ _____ and medical laboratory technicians perform diagnostic testing on blood, body fluids, and other types of specimens to assist the physician in obtaining a diagnosis.

10. _____ _____ provide direct patient care services under the supervision of licensed physicians. They are trained to diagnose and treat patients as directed by the physician.

11. _____ _____ are registered nurses who provide anesthetics to patients during care by surgeons, physicians, dentists, or other qualified healthcare professionals.

12. _____ _____ assist patients in regaining their mobility and improving their strength and range of motion, which may have been impaired by an accident or injury, or as a result of disease.

Chapter 2 Quiz

Name: _____

1. Which agency evaluates the quality of laboratory reports?

   a. OSHA

   b. CLIA

   c. CDC

2. Name a professional who works under the supervision of a medical technologist.

3. What type of registered nurse has advanced training to diagnose and treat common illnesses?

   a. anesthetist

   b. practitioner

   c. dietician

   d. practical

4. True or False: An occupational therapist works to help patients regain functions that will improve their quality of life.

5. A _____ treats life-threatening illnesses and supervises ambulance services.

6. _____ therapists are trained to use oxygen therapy and measure lung capacity.

7. True or False: Chiropractors write prescriptions.

8. The credentials DDS and DMD are used by

   _____.

9. The agency that inspects workplaces for safety is

   a. CDC

   b. OSHA

   c. DHHS

10. A way of prioritizing patients so that those with the most serious conditions receive care first is called

    a. case management

    b. accreditation

    c. triage

CHAPTER 3

The Medical Assisting Profession

Part I. Vocabulary

Directions: Define the following terms.

1. versatile _____

2. cross-training _____

3. phlebotomy _____

4. CEUs _____

Part II. The Profession

Describe how the medical assisting profession has evolved over the past 40 years.

_____

_____

_____

_____

_____

_____

_____

_____

Part III. Scope of Practice

A. Name the two major areas of medical assisting practice.

1. _____

2. _____

B. List some of the administrative duties of medical assistants.

1. _____
2. _____
3. _____

C. List some of the clinical duties of medical assistants.

1. _____
2. _____
3. _____

Which area do you think you enjoy most, administrative or clinical? Why?

_____
_____
_____
_____

Part IV. Educational Preparation

A. What are three educational levels in medical assisting?

1. _____
2. _____
3. _____

B. List six personal attributes that a student should show during his or her externship.

1. _____
2. _____
3. _____
4. _____
5. _____
6. _____

C. Name two reasons that continuing education is important to medical assistants.

1. _____
2. _____

Part V. Professional Appearance

A. Working with a partner, write a dress code for an office.

_____

_____

_____

_____

_____

_____

_____

_____

_____

_____

B. Locate the closest professional chapter for medical assistants. Record the name of the group, the date, and the location of their next meeting in your area.

_____

_____

_____

_____

Part VI. Professional Organizations

Directions: Complete the following sentences.

1. Gail uses the CMA credential behind her name. It stands for _____

_____ _____.

2. The CMA exam is offered by the _____.

3. Tom is looking for an accredited medical assisting program. The two agencies that accredit programs are _____ and _____.

4. The American Medical Technologists offer the _____ credential for graduates of accredited medical assisting programs who pass the exam.

Chapter 3 Quiz

Name: _____

1. The first national organization formed for medical assistants was:

   a. CAAHEP

   b. ABHES

   c. AMT

   d. AAMA

2. True or False: Both men and women can be equally successful as medical assistants.

3. True or False: Medical assistants may perform electrocardiograms and prepare patients for x-ray examinations.

4. True or False: Individuals working in the medical assisting field have a mandatory retirement age.

5. True or False: Most medical assisting positions are in hospitals.

6. True or False: The medical assisting student should treat the externship experience as if it were a probationary period for an actual job.

7. Which credential is **NOT** offered by the AMT?

   a. COLT

   b. RMA

   c. CMA

   d. RPT

8. True or False: Medical assistants always wear white uniforms.

CHAPTER 4

Professional Behavior in the Workplace

Part I. Vocabulary

Directions: Fill in the blanks with the appropriate vocabulary terms.

1. The nurse manager presents an employee-of-the-month certificate at staff meetings to boost employee _____.

2. Salaries are usually _____ with education and experience.

3. _____ means to intentionally put off doing something that should be done.

4. A medical assistant who is disrespectful to people in authority might be accused of

   _____.

5. When an employee volunteers to help in other departments, this shows _____.

6. Failure to follow preoperative instructions can be _____ to the patient's health.

7. _____ is characterized by conforming to ethical and technical standards.

Part II.

List the eight characteristics of the professional persona.

1. _____
2. _____
3. _____
4. _____
5. _____
6. _____
7. _____
8. _____

Part III.

List five deterrents to professionalism.

1. _____

2. _____

3. _____

4. _____

5. _____

Which of these five deterrents do you think will be the most difficult for you to deal with in the medical office?

_____

_____

Why? _____

_____

_____

_____

Part IV. _____

Directions: Your text lists four professional attributes. Rate yourself in each of the four areas by circling the appropriate statement.

Teamwork:	I need to improve.	I'm about average.	I'm a team player.
Time Management:	I need to improve.	I'm about average.	I am very organized.
Prioritizing:	I need to improve.	I'm about average.	This is one of my strengths.
Goal-Setting:	I need to improve.	I'm about average.	I'm goal-oriented.

Part V. _____

1. Karen seems to have trouble remembering exact doses of medications that were verbally ordered by Dr. Ross. How can she avoid this problem in the future?

_____

_____

_____

_____

_____

2. Karen works in the office lab. She is often asked questions about insurance and billing that she must refer to other personnel. How should Karen efficiently request information or assistance from other office personnel?

_____

_____

_____

_____

_____

3. The office manager has asked Karen to make sure her blood pressures are documented more legibly on the patient records. Why is neatness so important?

_____

_____

_____

_____

4. Karen and her fiancé broke up last week. How should she deal with personal stressors while she is in the workplace?

_____

_____

_____

_____

_____

_____

5. A patient needs to be scheduled for an outpatient endoscopic exam. When Karen gave the instruction sheet to the patient, she suspected that the patient was embarrassed because he could not read. How could Karen handle this situation?

_____

_____

_____

_____

_____

Chapter 4 Quiz

Name: _____

1. Which of the following words is misspelled?

   a. Characteristic

   b. Compitence

   c. Commensurate

2. True or False: Office politics are always negative.

3. _____ is to intentionally put off doing something that should be done.

   a. Initiative

   b. Procrastination

   c. Professionalism

   d. Discretion

4. True or False: Insubordination can be grounds for termination.

5. A _____, by definition, is talk or widely disseminated opinion with no discernible source or a statement that is not known to be true.

6. _____ is the process of working well with others to reach mutual goals.

7. True or False: Insubordination might be justified if you are asked to perform an illegal act.

8. Which of the following words is misspelled?

   a. Demeanor

   b. Discretion

   c. Disemminated

   d. Detrimental

CHAPTER 5

Interpersonal Skills and Human Behavior

Part I. Vocabulary

Directions: Use the appropriate vocabulary term from the text to complete each sentence.

1. Jill commented that the new office policies are confusing and _____.

2. Giving a patient an injection against his or her will could be considered _____.

3. Shane's remark was insulting and _____.

4. Whitney _____ denied leaving the narcotics cabinet unlocked.

5. With the increasing number of lawsuits, medical personnel can conclude that our society is quite

   _____.

6. Angry employees who are being terminated might be _____.

7. The notion that all physicians are male is an example of a _____.

8. Sayed uses positive _____ while he is training a new employee.

Part II.

Directions: Label the following questions as either open-ended or closed-ended.

1. _____ Are you taking blood pressure medicine?

2. _____ Are you allergic to aspirin?

3. _____ Would you tell me about your past surgeries?

4. _____ Do you have asthma?

5. _____ Do you smoke?

6. _____ Is your headache better today?

7. _____ Do you have hospitalization insurance?

8. _____ Do you want an afternoon appointment?

9. _____ How are you feeling today?

10. _____ Do you have trouble swallowing pills?

Part III.

Directions: Match the following defense mechanisms with the appropriate statements.

1. _____ "Everyone else is always late, so why am I getting written up for it?"

2. _____ "My husband can't have cancer. He is completely healthy."

3. _____ "I'd like to get better grades, but I can't find time to study."

4. _____ "I should phone my brother since our fight, but I just can't deal with that now."

5. _____ "Who are you to ask me that?"

6. _____ "I know I gained five pounds, Dr. George, but I exercised three times last week."

7. _____ "He only hits me because he is stressed at work."

8. _____ "I don't care what grade I made on the test because I am not going to pass the class anyway."

9. _____ "I have enough problems at work and don't need to come home to a nagging wife!"

10. _____ "I will never go to that restaurant again, because that is where my ex-husband proposed to me."

11. _____ "Of course it's a nice dress, if you like tents."

A. verbal aggression
B. sarcasm
C. rationalization
D. compensation
E. regression
F. repression
G. apathy
H. displacement
I. denial
J. avoidance
K. projection

Part IV.

Directions: List five barriers to communication.

1. _____
2. _____
3. _____
4. _____
5. _____

Part V. _____

Directions: Discuss the following scenarios as they relate to Maslow's hierarchy of needs.

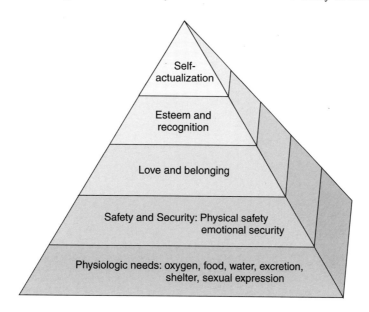

1. Kim is usually a good speller. However, her spelling grades have dropped since she was given a diagnosis of asthma.

_____

_____

_____

_____

2. In hazardous situations, paramedics are instructed to protect themselves before caring for patients.

_____

_____

_____

_____

3. Bill says that he could not pay attention during the staff meeting because he was distracted by the aroma from the large tray of pastries, which had been sent in by the sales representative from the drug company.

_____

_____

_____

_____

Chapter 5 Quiz

Name: _____

1. Which of the following words is misspelled?

    a. Litigious

    b. Paraphrasing

    c. Sarcasm

    d. Vehemently

2. _____ means easily aroused; tending to erupt in violence.

    a. Stereotype

    b. Vehemently

    c. Volatile

3. True or False: The description of the study of the phenomena of death and of psychological methods of coping with death is called *thanatology*.

4. True or False: According to Maslow, basic physiological needs must be met before higher level needs can be addressed.

5. _____ -ended questions are more likely to provide more information.

6. _____ is a sharp and often satirical response or ironic utterance designed to cut or give pain.

7. True or False: An older child who starts sucking his or her thumb during a stressful period might be demonstrating regressive behavior.

8. Which of the following defense mechanisms results in the inability to remember a painful event?

    a. Denial

    b. Repression

    c. Regression

    d. Apathy

CHAPTER 6

Medicine and Ethics

Part I. Vocabulary

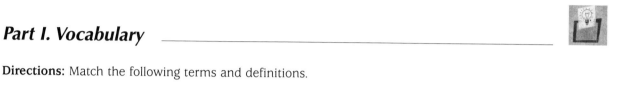

Directions: Match the following terms and definitions.

1. _____ Faithfulness to something to which one is bound by pledge or duty.

2. _____ The act of doing or producing good, especially performing acts of charity or kindness.

3. _____ The realm embracing property rights that belong to the community at large, are unprotected by copyright or patent, and are subject to appropriation by anyone.

4. _____ Refraining from the act of harming or committing evil.

5. _____ A devotion to, or conformity with, the truth.

6. _____ The act or practice of killing or permitting the death of hopelessly sick or injured individuals in a relatively painless way for reasons of mercy.

7. _____ Apportioning for a specific purpose or to particular persons or things.

A. euthanasia

B. allocating

C. veracity

D. fidelity

E. nonmaleficence

F. public domain

G. beneficence

Part II.

Directions: Label the following as nonmaleficence (N), veracity (V), fidelity (F), or beneficence (B).

1. _____ Melissa offers free blood pressure checks at her office on Wednesday afternoons.

2. _____ Dr. Parker insists that medical assistants check medications three times before administering them.

3. _____ Geri notified the office manager that she dropped the microscope while cleaning it.

4. _____ Joyce refuses to discuss office business with people outside work.

Part III.

A. **Directions:** List the five steps of ethical decision making.

a. _____

b. _____

c. _____

d. _____

e. _____

B. **Directions:** Indicate which statements are true (T) and which statements are false (F).

1. _____ A method of anonymous HIV testing in which a code is used instead of names to protect the confidentiality of the patient is illegal.

2. _____ Ramifications are consequences produced by a cause or following from a set of conditions.

3. _____ Clinical trials are research studies that test how well new medical treatments or other interventions work in the subjects, usually human beings.

Part IV.

Directions: Define each of the following ethical situations and describe some of the issues surrounding these topics.

Abortion

_____

_____

_____

_____

_____

Abuse

_____

_____

_____

_____

_____

_____

Allocation of Health Resources

_____
_____
_____
_____
_____

Artificial Insemination

_____
_____
_____
_____
_____

Surrogate Motherhood

_____
_____
_____
_____
_____

Human Cloning

_____
_____
_____
_____
_____

Genetic Counseling

_____
_____
_____
_____
_____

Physician-Assisted Suicide

_____
_____
_____
_____

Withholding or Withdrawing Life-Prolonging Treatment

_____
_____
_____
_____
_____

Organ Donation

_____
_____
_____
_____
_____

Capital Punishment

_____
_____
_____
_____
_____

HIV Testing

_____
_____
_____
_____
_____

Human Genome

_____
_____
_____
_____
_____

Fee-Splitting

_____

_____

_____

_____

_____

Part V. Workplace Applications _____

Scenario: You notice a co-worker giving out drug samples to someone without the permission of the physician.

Step One: Think about this situation and how you believe it should be handled. Record your ideas.

_____

_____

_____

_____

_____

Step Two: Pair up with a classmate and discuss your ideas. Record ideas on which you agree. List any new ideas. Note any items about which you disagree.

_____

_____

_____

_____

_____

Step Three: Share your ideas with your classmates. Make notes of any ideas that you did not think of before.

_____

_____

_____

_____

_____

_____

Chapter 6 Quiz

Name: _____

1. List four examples of ethical duties.

   a. _____

   b. _____

   c. _____

   d. _____

2. _____ deals with courtesy, customs, and manners.

3. The CEJA is part of the _____.

   a. AAMA

   b. AMA

   c. CMA

4. True or False: The access to genetic information prompts many concerns and presents ethical, legal, and moral questions.

5. True or False: The law requires that abuse be reported, and if a physician does not report abuse, his or her ethical standards have also been breached.

6. True or False: Confidentiality is one of the cardinal rules of the medical profession.

7. Define fee-splitting.

   _____

   _____

8. Define ghost surgery.

   _____

   _____

CHAPTER 7

Medicine and Law

Part I. Vocabulary

Directions: Supply the appropriate vocabulary words for the following definitions. Use the Word Find below for clues.

1. The hearing and determination of a cause in controversy by a person or persons either chosen by the parties involved or appointed under statutory authority. _____

2. An intentional, unlawful attempt to cause bodily injury to another by force. _____

3. An officer of some U.S. courts, usually serving as a messenger or usher, who keeps order at the request of the judge. _____

4. A coded delineation of the rules and regulations published in the *Federal Register* by the various departments and agencies of the federal government. _____

5. A sum imposed as punishment for an offense; a forfeiture or penalty paid to an injured party or the government in a civil or criminal action. _____

6. A willful and unlawful use of force or violence upon the person of another. _____

7. Of or relating to a judgment, the function of judging, the administration of justice, or the judiciary. _____

8. A binding custom or practice of a community; a rule of conduct or action prescribed or formally recognized as binding or enforceable by a controlling authority. _____

9. A major crime, such as murder, rape, or burglary; punishable by a more stringent sentence than that given for a misdemeanor. _____

10. A written defamatory statement or representation that conveys an unjustly unfavorable impression. _____

11. A writ or document commanding a person to appear in court under a penalty for failure to appear. _____

12. The finding or decision of a jury on a matter submitted to it in trial. _____

13. Marked by wisdom or judiciousness; shrewd in the management of practical affairs.

   _____

14. A court that sits in some cities and larger towns and that usually has civil and criminal jurisdiction over cases arising within the municipality. _____

15. A minor crime, as opposed to a felony, punishable by fine or imprisonment in a city or county jail rather than in a penitentiary. _____

Word Find

Directions: Use your answers above to find the terms.

```
M   F   I   N   E   T   L   U   A   S   S   A
I   T   M   J   U   D   I   C   I   A   L   N
S   N   U   B   K   A   B   T   E   G   C   S
D   O   N   W   I   P   E   C   T   B   E   A
E   I   I   C   B   R   L   I   O   E   C   N
M   T   C   F   A   U   U   D   Z   Y   L   O
E   A   I   F   T   D   K   R   R   N   A   E
A   G   P   I   T   E   M   E   A   O   W   P
N   E   A   L   E   N   T   V   T   L   I   B
O   L   L   L   R   T   N   T   W   E   D   U
R   L   Y   A   Y   R   F   C   X   F   R   S
S   A   R   B   I   T   R   A   T   I   O   N
```

Part II. _____

Directions: Complete the following lists and statements.

1. Name three categories of offenses in criminal law.

   a. _____

   b. _____

   c. _____

2. Name the three areas of civil law.

   a. _____

   b. _____

   c. _____

3. Describe the four elements of a contract.

   a. _____

   b. _____

   c. _____

   d. _____

4. To protect the physician against a lawsuit for _____, the details of the circumstances under which the physician is withdrawing from the case should be included in the patient's medical chart.

5. The letter of withdrawal does not have to specify a reason for withdrawal unless the physician so chooses, but it should state:

   a. _____

   b. _____

   c. _____

6. Letters of withdrawal are sent by _____.

Part III. _____

Directions: Use the appropriate terms to complete the sentences.

1. A _____ is usually taken in an attorney's office in the presence of a court reporter and is taken under oath.

2. A subpoena _____ _____ is a legally binding request to provide records or documents to be presented in court and is usually issued to the person considered the custodian of the records.

3. In a criminal case, the burden of proof is on the prosecution, which must prove guilt beyond any

   _____ _____.

4. Civil cases must be proven by a _____ _____ _____

   _____.

5. When a patient is injured as a result of a physician's negligence, the patient may initiate a

   malpractice lawsuit to recover financial _____.

6. The standard of prudent care and conduct is not defined by law but is left to the determination of

   a judge or jury, usually with the help of _____ _____.

Directions: For each case described below, discuss the Four D's of negligence.

1. A patient was given the wrong medication. There were no adverse effects. Which of the four D's is missing? Why?

   _____

   _____

   _____

   _____

2. A car wreck occurs at an intersection outside a doctor's office during normal business hours. Do the doctor and staff have a duty to provide direct care for the injured patients? Why?

   _____

   _____

   _____

   _____

3. A patient is treated for low back pain caused by a fall at the local grocery store. The patient sues the doctor because the pain is unresolved. Which of the four D's would be the most difficult for the plaintiff's attorney to prove? Why?

_____

_____

_____

_____

4. A medical assistant mislabeled a vial of blood that was sent to an outside laboratory. Because of this mistake, a child was given the wrong diagnosis and later died. The medical assistant, physician-employer, and the hospital that owns the practice were sued. The child's family was awarded a total of four million dollars. What type of damages are these? Why?

_____

_____

_____

_____

Part IV. Medical License

1. The purposes of the medical practice acts, established in every state by the beginning of the twentieth century, are to:

   • define what is included in the practice of medicine _____ _____

     _____;

   • govern the methods and _____ of licensure;

   • establish the grounds for _____ _____ _____ of license.

2. List three reasons a medical license can be suspended.

   a. _____

   b. _____

   c. _____

Extra for Experts

Directions: Research the following terms at the library or on the Internet. How do these issues relate to your practice as a medical assistant?

1. respondeat superior

2. vicarious liability

3. contributory negligence

Chapter 7 Quiz

Name: _____

1. A patient rolls up his sleeve for you to draw blood. Which type of consent is this?

   a. informed

   b. implied

   c. expressed

2. Name an agency that deals with administrative law.

3. In a medical malpractice suit, the doctor is usually the

   a. plaintiff

   b. attorney

   c. bailiff

   d. defendant

4. True or False: Consideration is an exchange of something of value, for example, money for the physician's time.

5. True or False: Schedule II drugs include narcotics and Ritalin.

6. A _____ of limitations is a period after which a lawsuit cannot be filed.

7. True or False: Informed consent includes knowledge of alternate treatments and risks.

8. An _____ _____ is a person younger than 18 or 21 years who can legally give consent.

9. The agency that regulates controlled substances is the

   a. FDA

   b. OSHA

   c. HIPPA

   d. DEA

10. Medical licensure can be obtained through

    a. examination

    b. reciprocity

    c. endorsement

    d. all of the above

CHAPTER 8

Computers in the Medical Office

Part I. Vocabulary

Directions: Use the appropriate vocabulary term from the text to fill in the blank.

1. Software programs designed to perform specific tasks. _____

2. The aspect of computer science that deals with computers taking on the attributes of humans. One such example is expert systems, which are capable of making decisions, such as software that is designed to help a physician make a diagnosis when given a set of symptoms. Game-playing programming and programs that are designed to recognize human language are other examples. _____ _____

3. American Standard Code for Information Interchange; a code representing English characters as numbers; each character is assigned a number from 0 to 127. _____

4. Any type of storage of files to prevent their loss in the event of hard disk failure. _____

5. A unit of data that contains eight binary digits. _____

6. A special form of high-speed storage, which can either be a part of the computer's main memory or can be a separate storage device. _____

7. A message that is sent to the web browser from the web server, which identifies users and can prepare custom web pages for them, possibly displaying their names on return to the site. _____

8. A symbol appearing on the monitor that shows where the next character to be typed will appear. _____

9. A collection of related files that serves as a foundation for retrieving information. _____

10. A magnetic surface that is capable of storing computer programs. _____

11. A term used to describe the sale and purchase of goods and services over the Internet; doing business over the Internet. _____

12. Communications transmitted via computer with a modem. _____

13. A design, similar to typesetting, for a set of characters. _____

14. To magnetically create tracks on a disk on which information will be stored, usually done by the manufacturer of the disk. _____

15. Approximately one billion bytes. _____

16. The readable paper copy or printout of information. _____

17. A common connection point for devices in a network containing multiple ports, often used to connect segments of a local area network (LAN). _____

18. Abbreviation for hyper text markup language, which is the language used to create documents for use on the Internet. _____

19. A picture, often on the desktop of a computer, which represents a program or object; by clicking on it, the user is directed to the program. _____

20. Information entered into and used by the computer. _____

21. An object-oriented high-level programming language commonly used and well-suited for the Internet. _____

22. Approximately one million bytes. _____

23. The measuring device for microprocessors, abbreviated MHz. _____

24. A device that allows information to be transmitted over phone lines, at speeds measured in bits per second (bps); short for modulator-demodulator. _____

25. The presentation of graphics, animation, video, sound, and text on a computer in an integrated way, or all at once. _____

26. Information that is processed by the computer and transmitted to a monitor, printer, or other device. _____

27. A device used to connect any number of local area networks (LANs), which communicate with other routers and determine the best route between any two hosts. _____

28. A device that reads text or illustrations on a printed page and can translate the information on that page into a form that the computer can understand. _____

29. Abbreviation for uniform resource locator; specifies the global address of documents or information on the Internet. _____

30. An artificial environment presented to a computer user, which simulates a real environment; the user often wears special gloves, earphones, and goggles to enhance the experience.

    _____ _____

31. A small and portable disk drive that is primarily used for backing up information and archiving computer files. It will hold the equivalent of about 70 floppy disks. _____

Part II. _____

A. **Directions:** Fill in the blanks.

  1. _____ is internal memory that contains a portion of the operating system and computer language. This is sometimes known as *main memory*.

2. _____ can be thought of as an internal scratch pad for the computer. It contains the program instructions and the data that are currently being processed, and it is normally erased when the power is shut off.

B. Workplace Applications

Directions: Describe two different ways to perform each task in a word-processing program.

1. Open a file.

_____

_____

2. Save a file.

_____

_____

3. Print a file.

_____

_____

4. Save a file under a different name.

_____

_____

5. Exit a program.

_____

_____

6. Cut and paste text.

_____

_____

7. Center text.

_____

_____

8. Bold text.

_____

_____

9. Insert a table.

_____

_____

10. Undo a mistake.

_____

_____

Part III.

A. **Directions:** Label each of the following as Input, Output, or Storage.

1. Mouse _____

2. Keyboard _____

3. Printer _____

4. Scanner _____

5. DVD _____

6. CD-ROM _____

7. Zip disk _____

8. Touch screen _____

9. Floppy disk _____

10. Modem _____

B. **Directions:** List seven ways that computers assist workers in medical offices.

1. _____

2. _____

3. _____

4. _____

5. _____

6. _____

7. _____

Part IV.

A. **Directions:** Give examples of each of the following.

1. Input _____

2. Processing _____

3. Storage _____

4. Output _____

B. **Directions:** Use an Internet search to visit various websites within the following domains; record the name of the agency and the URLs for the sites you find.

1. .com (for commercial businesses) _____

2. .org (for organizations, usually nonprofit) _____

3. .edu (for educational institutions) _____

4. .gov (for governmental agencies) _____

5. .net (for network organizations) _____

C. Visit a local store that sells computers or use a newspaper to examine a particular computer that is being sold. Answer the following questions.

1. How much RAM and ROM does the system have? _____

2. What is the clock speed? _____

3. What type of data storage is available? _____

4. What is the baud rate of the modem? _____

5. What software comes with the system? _____

6. Is a printer included? If so, what type? _____

7. Document the name of the store and price of the system. _____

D. **Directions:** Examine the work setting below. Label the numbered items as lighting, work surface, mouse, monitors, keyboards, storage and files, or adjustable chairs.

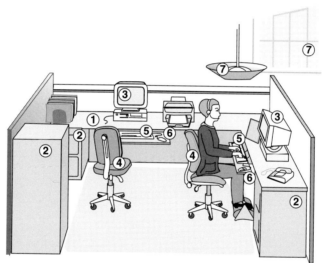

Ergonomic environment of an HIM department. (Redrawn from Gaylor L: The Administrative Dental Assistant, Philadelphia, WB, Saunders, 2000, p. 290.) (From Davis N, LaCour M: *Introduction to health information technology,* Philadelphia, 2002, WB Saunders.)

1. _____

2. _____

3. _____

4. _____

5. _____

6. _____

7. _____

CHAPTER 9

Telephone Technique

Part I. Vocabulary

Directions: Match the following terms and definitions.

1. _____ The quality or state of being clear.

2. _____ Having adequate abilities or qualilties; having the capacity to function or perform in a certain way.

3. _____ To foster the growth of; to improve by labor, care, or study.

4. _____ The choice of words especially with regard to clearness, correctness, or effectiveness.

5. _____ To utter articulate, clear sounds.

6. _____ A change in pitch or loudness of the voice.

7. _____ Consistent; not changing or capable of change.

8. _____ The technical terminology or characteristic idiom of a particular group or special activity.

9. _____ Performing multiple tasks at one time.

10. _____ The property of a sound and especially a musical tone that is determined by the frequency of the waves producing it; the highness or lowness of sound.

11. _____ Individual or company that provides medical care and services to the patient or the public.

12. _____ An expression of greeting, good will, or courtesy by words or gestures.

13. _____ Something that shields, protects, or hides; to select or eliminate through a screening process.

14. _____ Medical abbreviation for immediately; at this moment.

15. _____ Having a keen sense of what to do or say to maintain good relations with others or avoid offense.

16. _____ Tiresome because of length or dullness.

A. jargon

B. clarity

C. stat

D. competence

E. invariable

F. enunciate

G. diction

H. cultivate

I. inflection

J. tedious

K. screen

L. tactful

M. multitasking

N. provider

O. salutation

P. pitch

Part II.

Directions: Practice taking telephone messages on the forms provided.

1. Mr. Ross called today at 10:15 AM to get his prescription for Prozac refilled at Cunningham Drugs, phone 555-1372. The patient's phone number is 555-4573. He is allergic to penicillin.

2. Mrs. Garrett from Blue Cross called at 2:00 PM today to discuss employee benefits with your office manager. She would like for her to return the call before 5:00 PM today. Her extension is #415.

3. The Upstate Lab called at 9:35 AM to report a panic potassium level of 3.0 for a patient named Laura Williams. Dr. Lee is to be notified immediately.

Part III.

A. **Directions:** Fill in the blanks with the correct times.

When it is noon Pacific time, it is _____ PM Eastern time. Plan to make calls from San

Francisco to a business or professional office in New York no later than _____ PM.

When it is 2:00 PM on the West Coast, it is _____ PM on the East Coast.

B. **Directions:** List four ways to end a call.

1. _____

2. _____

3. _____

4. _____

C. **Directions:** Describe four rules for cell phone use.

1. _____

2. _____

3. _____

4. _____

MESSAGE FROM

For Dr.	Name of Caller	Ref. to pt.	Patient	Pt. Age	Pt. Temp.	Message Date	Message Time AM PM	Urgent ❑ Yes ❑ No

Message: Allergies

Respond to Phone #	Best Time to Call AM PM	Pharmacy Name / #	Patient's Chart Attached ❑ Yes ❑ No	Patient's chart #	Initials

DOCTOR - STAFF RESPONSE

Doctor's / Staff Orders / Follow-up Action

	Call Back ❑ Yes ❑ No	Chart. Mes. ❑ Yes ❑ No	Follow-up Date / /	Follow-up Completed-Date/Time / / AM PM	Response By:

Product # 78-9156-Pkg, #78-9157-Pads, Bibbero Systems, Inc., Petaluma, CA. To order, call toll free 800-BIBBERO (800 242-2376) OR FAX 800-242-9330.

MESSAGE FROM

For Dr.	Name of Caller	Ref. to pt.	Patient	Pt. Age	Pt. Temp.	Message Date	Message Time AM PM	Urgent ❑ Yes ❑ No

Message: Allergies

Respond to Phone #	Best Time to Call AM PM	Pharmacy Name / #	Patient's Chart Attached ❑ Yes ❑ No	Patient's chart #	Initials

DOCTOR - STAFF RESPONSE

Doctor's / Staff Orders / Follow-up Action

	Call Back ❑ Yes ❑ No	Chart. Mes. ❑ Yes ❑ No	Follow-up Date / /	Follow-up Completed-Date/Time / / AM PM	Response By:

Product # 78-9156-Pkg, #78-9157-Pads, Bibbero Systems, Inc., Petaluma, CA. To order, call toll free 800-BIBBERO (800 242-2376) OR FAX 800-242-9330.

MESSAGE FROM

For Dr.	Name of Caller	Ref. to pt.	Patient	Pt. Age	Pt. Temp.	Message Date	Message Time AM PM	Urgent ❑ Yes ❑ No

Message: Allergies

Respond to Phone #	Best Time to Call AM PM	Pharmacy Name / #	Patient's Chart Attached ❑ Yes ❑ No	Patient's chart #	Initials

DOCTOR - STAFF RESPONSE

Doctor's / Staff Orders / Follow-up Action

	Call Back ❑ Yes ❑ No	Chart. Mes. ❑ Yes ❑ No	Follow-up Date / /	Follow-up Completed-Date/Time / / AM PM	Response By:

Product # 78-9156-Pkg, #78-9157-Pads, Bibbero Systems, Inc., Petaluma, CA. To order, call toll free 800-BIBBERO (800 242-2376) OR FAX 800-242-9330.

Message forms. Courtesy of Bibbero Systems.

Part IV.

Your office manager is discussing revisions on a report that she is having you prepare for a staff meeting. You are also covering the telephone for a co-worker. The phone starts ringing. How will you handle this situation?

_____

_____

_____

_____

_____

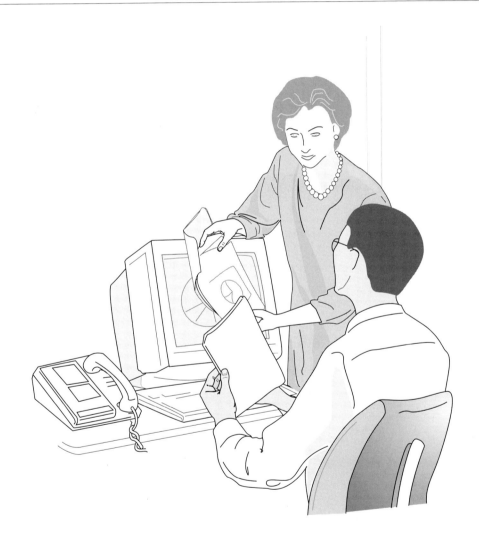

CHAPTER 10

Scheduling Appointments

Part I. Vocabulary

Directions: Fill in the blanks with the appropriate vocabulary words.

1. To break down or throw into disorder. _____

2. Patients who are returning to the office who have previously seen the physician.

   _____ _____

3. A situation requiring haste or caution; a means of achieving a particular end. _____

4. Essential; being an indispensable part of a whole. _____

5. A two-way communication; mutual or reciprocal action or influence. _____

6. Coming and going at intervals; not continuous. _____

7. Length of time between events. _____

8. Something in which a thing originates, develops, takes shape, or is contained; a base on which to build. _____

9. A person who fails to keep an appointment without giving advance notice. _____

10. Something that is necessary to achieve an end or to carry out a function. _____

11. Competency as a result of training or practice. _____

12. Relating to a combination of social and economic factors. _____

13. Responding to requests for immediate care and treatment after the urgency of the need has been evaluated and the treatment has been prioritized. _____

Part II.

A. **Directions:** Practice completing appointment reminder cards on the forms provided.

   1. Joey McGothlin has an appointment for Aug 23, 20XX, at 3 PM with Dr. Bachlet.

   2. Jennifer Dahlin has an appointment for Sept 10, 20XX, at 1 PM with Dr. Shaw.

Appointment reminder cards.

B. **Directions:** Prepare an appointment book page for Monday, Oct 13, by using the form provided on p. 59.

1. Drs. Lawler and Hughes have hospital rounds from 8 to 9 AM.

2. Dr. Lupez is seeing patients at a satellite office from 8 AM to noon.

3. Lunch is from noon to 1 PM.

4. Dr. Lawler has a 4 PM meeting at the hospital.

5. Dr. Hughes and Dr. Lupez prefer to have some time from 3:15 to 3:30 PM to catch up on dictation.

C. **Directions:** Schedule the following patients by using the form on p. 59.

1. Tracey and Keith Jones would like an appointment with Dr. Lawler right before lunch. Both are new patient physicals. Husband and wife would like to come at same time to discuss family planning.

2. John Edgar, Lydia Perry, and June Trayner—all established patients—need physicals for work performed by Dr. Lupez.

4. Wayne Harris, physical, new patient, as early as possible with Dr. Lawler.

5. Lucy Fraser, recheck with Dr. Hughes. Can be there by 4 PM right after picking up children from school.

6. Dr. Hughes has three rechecks for Monday morning: Asa Nordholm, Carrie Jones, and Wilma Stevens.

7. Talia Perez called and is having trouble with new blood pressure medicine. The only time she can get off work is at 2:15 PM.

8. Dr. Lawler has three rechecks: Ella Jones, Fred Linstra, and Mary Higgins.

9. Winston Hill is an established patient coming in for an annual physical with Dr. Lawler. His neighbor can drive him to the office around 2 PM.

10. Einar Rosen, an established patient, needs a physical with Dr. Hughes around 10:15 PM.

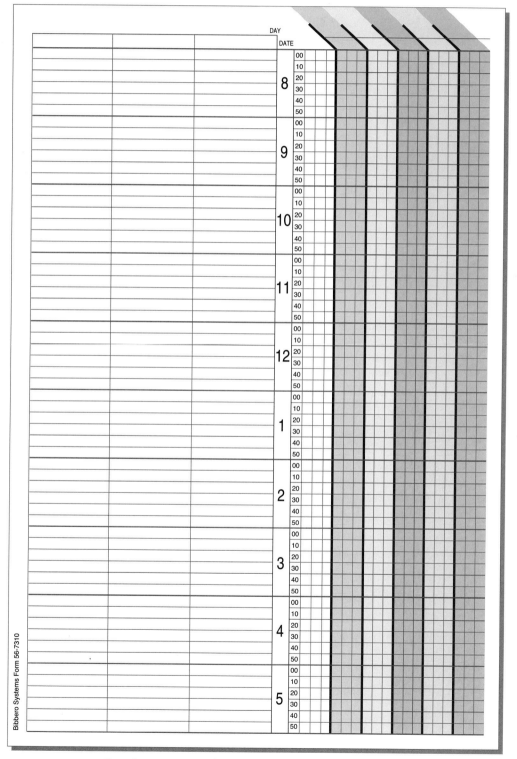

Sample appointment book page. Courtesy Bibbero Systems.

Part III.

A. **Directions:** List three items that must be considered when appointments are scheduled.

1. _____

2. _____

3. _____

B. **Directions:** List four basic features to consider in choosing an appointment book.

1. _____

2. _____

3. _____

4. _____

Part IV.

Directions: Briefly describe each system of scheduling. What are your concerns about each?

Scheduled Appointments

_____
_____
_____

Open Office Hours

_____
_____
_____

Flexible Office Hours

_____
_____
_____

Wave Scheduling

_____
_____
_____

Modified Wave Scheduling

_____
_____
_____

Double Booking

_____
_____
_____

Grouping Procedures

_____
_____
_____

Advance Booking

_____
_____
_____

CHAPTER 11

Patient Reception and Processing

Part I. Vocabulary

Directions: Define the following:

1. Amenity

2. Intercom

3. Progress notes

4. Demographic

Part II.

Directions: Correct the misspelled words.

1. Fevrent
2. Flaged
3. Harmoneous
4. Immigrent
5. Perseption
6. Phonitec
7. Sequencially

Part III.

A. Visit several reception areas for local banks, hospitals, doctors' offices, or even your school. Record your impressions in the table below.

Location				
Cleanliness				
Colors				
Seating				
Lighting				
Comfort				
Amenities				
Noise				

B. Paige is getting ready for the next workday. What is the first step in preparing for patient arrival? What will she need to look at to complete this task?

_____

_____

_____

_____

C. What is another task that she could complete the evening before?

_____

_____

_____

Part IV.

A. What are your thoughts and concerns regarding patient check-in?

_____

_____

_____

B. On the blank letterhead provided on p. 66, design your own registration form.

C. List several routine tasks for closing an office.

_____

_____

_____

_____

D. How do you feel about asking for payments and copayments?

_____

_____

_____

_____

Blackburn Primary Care Associates
1990 Turquoise Drive
Blackburn, WI 54937
(555) 555-1234

E. With a partner, role play. Pretend you are interviewing a patient named Ivan Shapiro. Find out more about his chest pain, what medicines he is taking, and his past illnesses. Document his responses on the health history form provided.

Case One, Form 3

ANDRUS/CLINI-REC® HEALTH HISTORY QUESTIONNAIRE

Chart No. _____

Identification Information

Today's Date _____

Name __Shapiro, Ivan_____   Date of Birth __3/6/45__

Occupation __Carpenter_____   Marital Status __Married__

PART A – PRESENT HEALTH HISTORY

I. CURRENT MEDICAL PROBLEMS

Please list the medical problems for which you came to see the doctor. About when did they begin?

Problems	Date Began
Chest pain when exercising	

What concerns you most about these problems?

If you are being treated for any other illness or medical problems by another physician, please describe the problems and write the name of the physician or medical facility treating you.

Illness or Medical Problem	Physician or Medical Facility	City

II. MEDICATIONS

Please list all medications you are now taking, including those you buy without a doctor's prescription (such as aspirin, cold tablets or vitamin supplements).

III. ALLERGIES AND SENSITIVITIES

List anything that you are allergic to such as certain foods, medications, dust, chemicals or soaps, household items, pollens, bee stings, etc., and indicate how each affects you.

Allergic To:	Effect	Allergic To:	Effect
Penicillin	Hives		

IV. GENERAL HEALTH, ATTITUDE AND HABITS

How is your overall health now?	Health now:	Poor ____	Fair ____	Good _X_	Excellent ____
How has it been most of your life?	Health has been:	Poor ____	Fair ____	Good _X_	Excellent ____

In the past year:

Has your appetite changed?	Appetite:	Decreased ____	Increased ____	Stayed same _X_
Has your weight changed?	Weight:	Lost ____ lbs.	Gained _10_ lbs.	No change ____
Are you thirsty much of the time?	Thirsty:	No _X_	Yes ____	
Has your overall 'pep' changed?	Pep:	Decreased ____	Increased ____	Stayed same _X_
Do you usually have trouble sleeping?	Trouble sleeping:	No ____	Yes _X_	
How much do you exercise?	Exercise:	Little or none ____	Less than I need ____	All I need _X_
Do you smoke?	Smokes:	No _X_	Yes ____	If yes, how many years? ____
How many each day?		____ Cigarettes	____ Cigars	____ Pipesfull
Have you ever smoked?	Smoked:	No ____	Yes _X_	If yes, how many years? _15_
How many each day?		_20_ Cigarettes	____ Cigars	____ Pipesfull
Do you drink alcoholic beverages?	Alcohol:	No ____ Yes _X_	I drink ____ Beers ____ Glasses of wine ____ Drinks of hard liquor - per day _Socially_	
Have you ever had a problem with alcohol?	Prior problem:	No _X_	Yes ____	
How much coffee or tea do you usually drink?	Coffee/Tea:	_2_ cups of coffee or tea a day		
Do you regularly wear seatbelts?	Seatbelts:	No ____	Yes _X_	

DO YOU:	Rarely/Never	Occasionally	Frequently	DO YOU:	Rarely/Never	Occasionally	Frequently
Feel nervous?	X			Ever feel like committing suicide?	X		
Feel depressed?	X						
Find it hard to make decisions?	X			Feel bored with your life?	X		
Lose your temper?		X		Use marijuana?	X		
Worry a lot?	X			Use "hard drugs"?	X		
Tire easily?		X		Do you want to talk to the doctor about a personal matter? No _X_ Yes ____			
Have trouble relaxing?		X					
Have any sexual problems?	X						

Created and Developed by "Medical Economics" Professional Systems
Copyright © 1979, 1983 Bibbero Systems International, Inc.

STOCK NO. 19-742-4   8/95   Page 1

Courtesy of Bibbero Systems, Inc., Petaluma, California.

Health history questionnaire

Case One, Form 3   **PART A – PRESENT HEALTH HISTORY (continued)**

IV. GENERAL HEALTH, ATTITUDE AND HABITS (continued)

Have you recently had any changes in your: If yes, please explain:

Marital status?	No __X__ Yes _____	
Job or work?	No _____ Yes __X__	Self employed
Residence?	No _____ Yes __X__	Moved from LA CA
Financial status?	No __X__ Yes _____	

Are you having any legal problems
or trouble with the law?   No __X__ Yes _____

PART B – PAST HISTORY

I. FAMILY HEALTH

Please give the following information about your immediate family:

Relationship	Age, if Living	Age At Death	State of Health Or Cause of Death
Father	_____	78	Lung cancer
Mother		45	Heart disease
Brothers and Sisters	38		good
	_____	_____	_____
	_____	_____	_____
Spouse	51	_____	good
Children	22	_____	good
	25	_____	good

Have any **blood relatives** had any of the following illnesses?
If so, indicate relationship (mother, brother, etc.)

Illness	Family Members
Asthma	_____
Diabetes	_____
Cancer	Father
Blood Disease	_____
Glaucoma	_____
Epilepsy	_____
Rheumatoid Arthritis	Aunt
Tuberculosis	_____
Gout	_____
High Blood Pressure	Mother
Heart Disease	Mother
Mental Problems	_____
Suicide	_____
Stroke	Grandmother
Alcoholism	_____
Rheumatic Fever	_____

II. HOSPITALIZATIONS, SURGERIES, INJURIES

Please list all times you have been hospitalized, operated on, or seriously injured.

Year	Operation, Illness, Injury	Hospital and City
1990	Appendix removed	LA CA
_____	_____	_____
_____	_____	_____

III. ILLNESS AND MEDICAL PROBLEMS

Please mark with an (X) any of the following illnesses and medical problems you have or have had and indicate the year when each started. If you are not certain when an illness started, write down an approximate year.

Illness	(x)	(Year)	Illness	(x)	(Year)
Eye or eye lid infection	___	_____	Hernia	___	_____
Glaucoma	___	_____	Hemorrhoids	___	_____
Other eye problems	___	_____	Kidney or bladder disease	___	_____
Ear trouble	___	_____	Prostate problem (male only)	___	_____
Deafness or decreased hearing	___	_____	Mental problems	___	_____
Thyroid trouble	___	_____	Headaches	___	_____
Strep throat	___	_____	Head injury	___	_____
Bronchitis	___	_____	Stroke	___	_____
Emphysema	___	_____	Convulsions, seizures	___	_____
Pneumonia	___	_____	Arthritis	___	_____
Allergies, asthma or hay fever	___	_____	Gout	___	_____
Tuberculosis	___	_____	Cancer or tumor	___	_____
Other lung problems	___	_____	Bleeding tendency	___	_____
High blood pressure	___	_____	Diabetes	___	_____
Heart attack	___	_____	Measles/Rubeola	___	_____
High cholesterol	___	_____	German measles/Rubella	___	_____
Arteriosclerosis			Polio	___	_____
(Hardening of arteries)	___	_____	Mumps	___	_____
Heart murmur	___	_____	Scarlet fever	___	_____
Other heart condition	___	_____	Chicken pox	___	_____
Stomach/duodenal ulcer	___	_____	Mononucleosis	___	_____
Diverticulosis	___	_____	Eczema	___	_____
Colitis	___	_____	Psoriasis	___	_____
Other bowel problems	___	_____	Venereal disease	___	_____
Hepatitis	___	_____	Genital herpes	___	_____
Liver trouble	___	_____	HIV test	___	_____
Gallbladder trouble	___	_____	AIDS	___	_____

(Vertical left margin: C O N F I D E N T I A L)

© 1979, 1983 Bibbero Systems International, Inc.   To Order Call:800-BIBBERO (800 242-2376)
Or Fax: (800 242-9330)
(REV. 8/95)
STOCK NO. 19-742-4   8/95

Page 2

Health history questionnaire—cont'd

CHAPTER 12

Written Communications and Mail Processing

Part I. Vocabulary

Directions: Define the following.

1. Watermark _____

2. Portfolio _____

3. Ream _____

4. Archived _____

5. Flush _____

Part II.

A. **Directions:** Label the parts of the letter provided on p. 70 and write in how many lines are between each section.

B. **Directions:** Correct the following envelope addresses.

Dr. Jim Smith, MD
301 Wst Hughes Str.
CHICAGO, ILL 54321

CINDY JOHNSON
1467 E GREEN ST
SUITE 409
BAYFIELD, GEORGIA 12345

Jose Kelley
Memorial Lane #321
West columbia, FL
98765

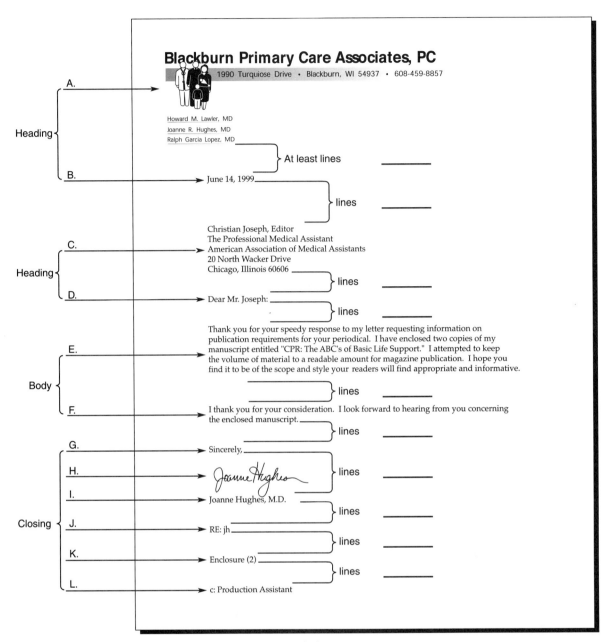

Blackburn Primary Care Associates, PC

1990 Turquiose Drive • Blackburn, WI 54937 • 608-459-8857

Heading

A.

Howard M. Lawler, MD
Joanne R. Hughes, MD
Ralph Garcia Lopez, MD

At least ____ lines   _____

B.

June 14, 1999   ____ lines   _____

Heading

C.

Christian Joseph, Editor
The Professional Medical Assistant
American Association of Medical Assistants
20 North Wacker Drive
Chicago, Illinois 60606   ____ lines   _____

D.

Dear Mr. Joseph: ____ lines   _____

Body

E.

Thank you for your speedy response to my letter requesting information on publication requirements for your periodical. I have enclosed two copies of my manuscript entitled "CPR: The ABC's of Basic Life Support." I attempted to keep the volume of material to a readable amount for magazine publication. I hope you find it to be of the scope and style your readers will find appropriate and informative.

____ lines   _____

F.

I thank you for your consideration. I look forward to hearing from you concerning the enclosed manuscript.   ____ lines   _____

Closing

G.

Sincerely,

H.

Joanne Hughes   ____ lines   _____

I.

Joanne Hughes, M.D.   ____ lines   _____

J.

RE: jh   ____ lines   _____

K.

Enclosure (2)   ____ lines   _____

L.

c: Production Assistant

Sample letter

Part III. _____

A. List several pieces of equipment used for written correspondence.

_____

_____

_____

B. List some of the supplies used for written correspondence.

_____

_____

_____

_____

C. What is standard letter-size paper? _____

D. List and describe three types of envelopes used in the office setting. Describe how letters are folded to fit each one.

_____

_____

_____

_____

_____

_____

_____

_____

E. List four parts of a letter.

1. _____

2. _____

3. _____

4. _____

F. Name three items that should be on a continuation page.

1. _____

2. _____

3. _____

Part IV. _____

A. What is the difference between registered and certified mail?

_____

_____

_____

_____

B. On the blank letterhead provided, practice writing a letter in block style.

Blackburn Primary Care Associates
1990 Turquoise Drive
Blackburn, WI 54937
(555) 555-1234

C. Practice writing a memo on the form provided.

MEMORANDUM

Date:

To:

From:

Subject:

Sample form for memo.

D. Design a fax cover sheet on the form provided on p. 74.

From:

To:

Phone Number:

Fax Number:

Blackburn Primary Care Associates
1990 Turquoise Drive
Blackburn, WI 54937
(555) 555-1234

CHAPTER 13

Medical Records Management

Part I. Vocabulary

Directions: Insert the correct vocabulary word.

1. _____ Systems made up of combinations of letters and numbers.

2. _____ A formal examination of an organization's or individual's accounts or financial situation; a methodical examination and review.

3. _____ To make greater, more numerous, larger, or more intense.

4. _____ A heading, title, or subtitle under which records are filed.

5. _____ Of, relating to, or arranged in or according to the order of time.

6. _____ The act or manner of uttering words to be transcribed.

7. _____ _____ _____ A filing system in which materials can be located without consulting an intermediary source of reference.

8. _____ _____ _____ A filing system in which an intermediary source of reference, such as a card file, must be consulted to locate specific files.

9. _____ A film bearing a photographic record on a reduced scale of printed or other graphic matter.

10. _____ Information that is gathered by watching or observing a patient.

11. _____ A method of filing whereby one report is laid on top of the older report, resembling the shingles of a roof.

12. _____ Information that is gained by questioning the patient or taken from a form.

13. _____ A chronological file used as a reminder that something must be taken care of on a certain date.

14. _____ To make a written copy of, either in longhand or by machine.

Part II.

A. **Directions:** Indicate where you would look for information on the following patients.

1. Veronica Marcengill _____

2. Jennings Carter _____

3. Madison Jennings _____

4. Mary Lismore-Golden _____

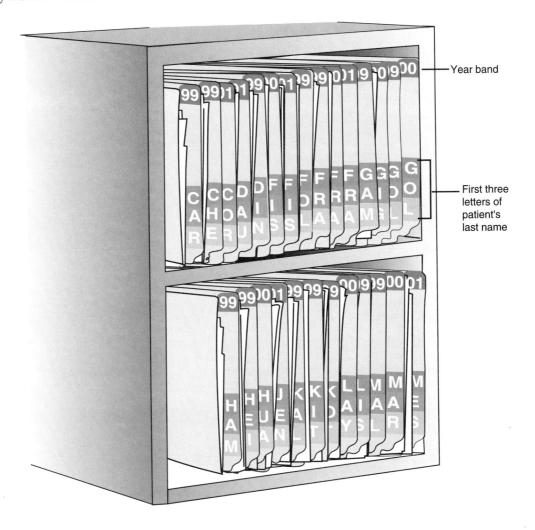

Year band

First three letters of patient's last name

B. Indicate where you would file the records for the following patients.

1. Mary Smith _____

2. Mike Smith _____

3. Ann Davis-Adams _____

4. Joe Brown, Jr. _____

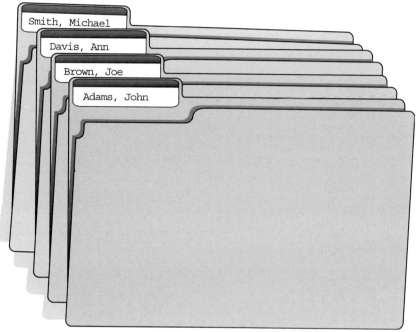

File folder labeling showing top tabs.

Part III. _____

A. **Directions:** Examine the file folder on p. 78. What information is available on the folder? What is the major advantage of this filing system?

_____

_____

_____

_____

_____

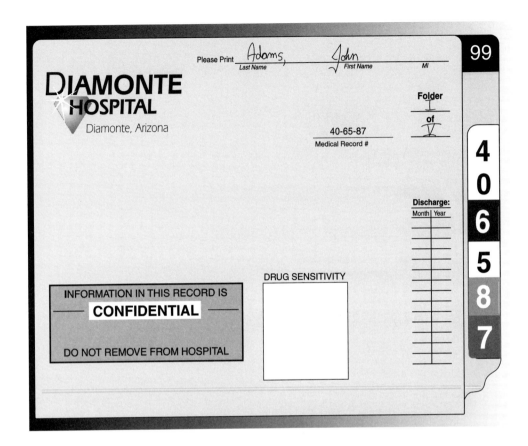

B. **Directions:** Label each type of filing system. What are some of the advantages and disadvantages?

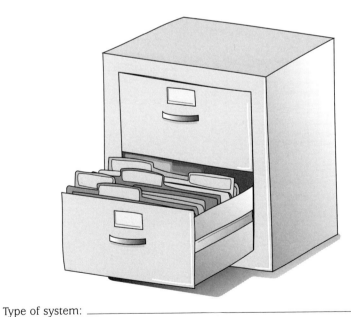

Type of system: _____.

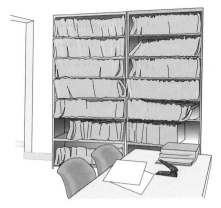

Type of system: _____.

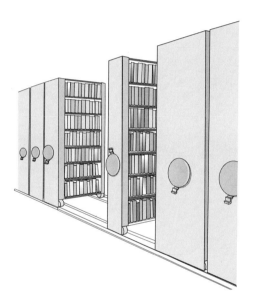

Type of system: _____.

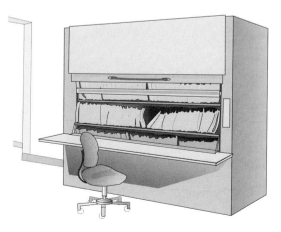

Type of system: _____.

Part IV.

A. **Directions:** Research various information storage systems. For each type that is pictured, list advantages and disadvantages.

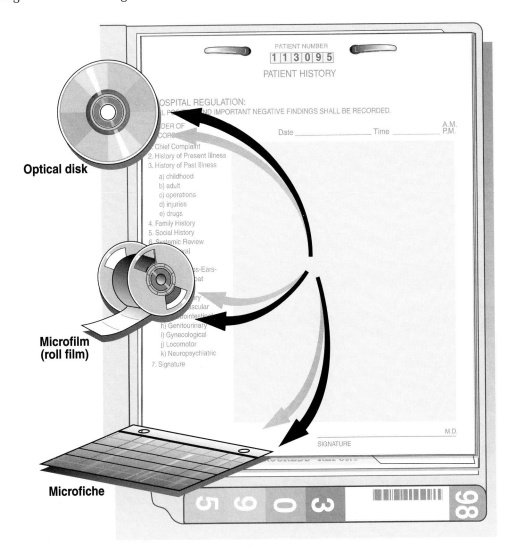

Disk: _____

_____

_____

Microfilm: _____

_____

_____

Microfiche: _____

_____

_____

B. Identify the item in the picture below. What are the advantages of using this item?

_____

_____

_____

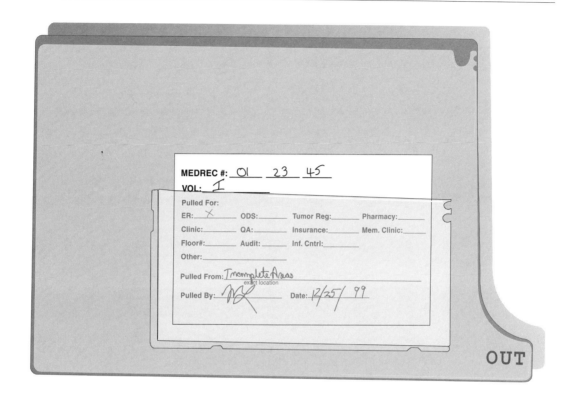

MEDREC #: _Ol_ _23_ _45_

VOL: _I_

Pulled For:

ER: _X_   ODS:_____   Tumor Reg:_____   Pharmacy:_____

Clinic:_____   QA:_____   Insurance:_____   Mem. Clinic:_____

Floor#:_____   Audit:_____   Inf. Cntrl:_____

Other:_____

Pulled From: _Incomplete Areas_
                         exact location

Pulled By: _____   Date: _12/25/ 99_

OUT

CHAPTER 14

Professional Fees, Billing, and Collecting

Part I. Vocabulary

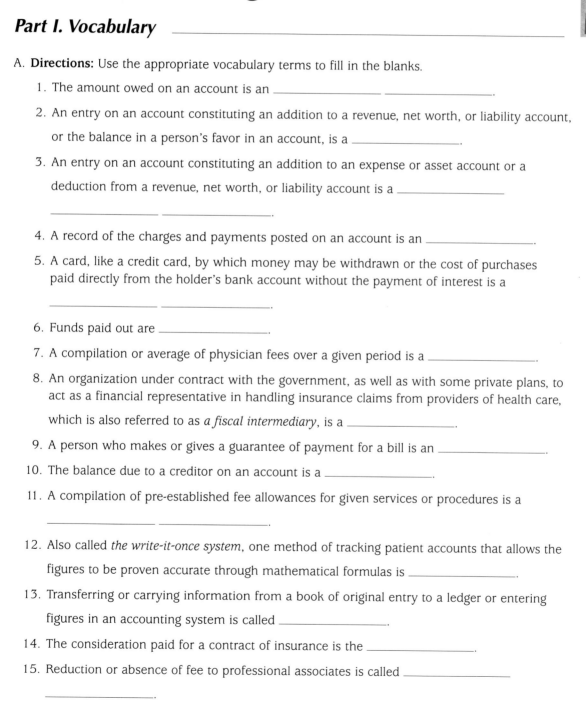

A. **Directions:** Use the appropriate vocabulary terms to fill in the blanks.

1. The amount owed on an account is an _____ _____.

2. An entry on an account constituting an addition to a revenue, net worth, or liability account, or the balance in a person's favor in an account, is a _____.

3. An entry on an account constituting an addition to an expense or asset account or a deduction from a revenue, net worth, or liability account is a _____ _____ _____.

4. A record of the charges and payments posted on an account is an _____.

5. A card, like a credit card, by which money may be withdrawn or the cost of purchases paid directly from the holder's bank account without the payment of interest is a _____ _____.

6. Funds paid out are _____.

7. A compilation or average of physician fees over a given period is a _____.

8. An organization under contract with the government, as well as with some private plans, to act as a financial representative in handling insurance claims from providers of health care, which is also referred to as *a fiscal intermediary*, is a _____.

9. A person who makes or gives a guarantee of payment for a bill is an _____.

10. The balance due to a creditor on an account is a _____.

11. A compilation of pre-established fee allowances for given services or procedures is a _____ _____.

12. Also called *the write-it-once system*, one method of tracking patient accounts that allows the figures to be proven accurate through mathematical formulas is _____.

13. Transferring or carrying information from a book of original entry to a ledger or entering figures in an accounting system is called _____.

14. The consideration paid for a contract of insurance is the _____.

15. Reduction or absence of fee to professional associates is called _____ _____.

16. Amounts paid on patient accounts are _____. Total monies received on accounts are _____.

17. Someone other than the patient, spouse, or parent who is responsible for paying all or part of the patient's medical costs is a _____ _____.

18. An exchange or transfer of goods, services, or funds is a _____.

B. **Directions:** Define the following.

Usual _____

Customary _____

Reasonable _____

C. **Directions:** Match the following terms and definitions.

1. _____ On the left, is used for entering charges, is sometimes called the *charge column*.

2. _____ To the right, sometimes headed "Paid," is used for entering payments received.

3. _____ On the far right, is used for recording the differences between the debit and credit columns.

4. _____ Is available in some systems and is used for entering professional discounts, write-offs, and disallowances.

A. Adjustment column

B. Debit column

C. Balance column

D. Credit column

D. **Directions:** List two steps in dealing with a returned check.

1. _____

2. _____

E. **Directions:** List the three basic forms in a pegboard system.

1. _____

2. _____

3. _____

Part II. _____

Directions: Examine the fee schedule on p. 85, and answer the following questions.

1. What is the charge for a consultation? _____

2. What is the charge for a 99203? _____

3. Why is the charge different for a 99213? _____

4. What is the most expensive procedure on the list? _____

   CPT Code_____

5. Which injection is more expensive, insulin or vitamin B_{12}? _____

FEE SCHEDULE

BLACKBURN PRIMARY CARE ASSOCIATES, PC
1990 Turquiose Drive
Blackburn, WI 54937
608-459-8857

Federal Tax ID Number: 00-0000000

BCBS Group Number: 14982
Medicare Group Number: 14982

OFFICE VISIT, NEW PATIENT

Focused, 99201	$45.00
Expanded, 99202	$55.00
Intermediate, 99203	$60.00
Extended, 99204	$95.00
Comprehensive, 99205	$195.00
Consultation, 99245	$250.00

OFFICE VISIT, ESTABLISHED PATIENT

Minimal, 99211	$40.00
Focused, 99212	$48.00
Intermediate, 99213	$55.00
Extended, 99214	$65.00
Comprehensive, 99215	$195.00

OFFICE PROCEDURES

EKG, 12 lead, 93000	$55.00
Stress EKG, Treadmill, 93015	$295.00
Sigmoidoscopy, Flex; 45330	$145.00
Spirometry, 94010	$50.00
Cerumen Removal, 69210	$40.00
Collection & Handling	
Lab Specimen, 99000	$9.00
Venipuncture, 35415	$9.00
Urinalysis, 81000	$20.00
Urinalysis, 81002 (Dip Only)	$12.00
Influenza Injection, 90724	$20.00
Pneumococcal Injection, 90732	$20.00
Oral Polio, 90712	$15.00
DTaP, 90700	$20.00
Tetanus Toxoid, 90703	$15.00
MMR, 90707	$25.00
HIB, 90737	$20.00
Hepatitis B, newborn to age 11 years, 90744	$60.00
Hepatitis B, 11-19 years, 90745	$60.00
Hepatitis B, 20 years and above 90746	$60.00
Intramuscular Injection, 90788	
Penicillin	$30.00
Cephtriaxone	$25.00
Solu-Medrol	$23.00
Vitamin B-12	$13.00
Subcutaneous Injection, 90782	
Epinephrine	$18.00
Susphrine	$25.00
Insulin, U-100	$15.00

COMMON DIAGNOSTIC CODES

Ischemic Heart Disease	414.9
w/o myocardial infarction	411.89
w/coronary occlusion	411.81
Hypertension, Malignant	401.0
Benign	401.1
Unspecified	401.9
w/congest. heart failure	402.91
Asthma, Bronchial	493.9
w/ COPD	493.2
allergic, w/ S.A.	493.91
allergic, w/o S.A.	493.90
Kyphosis	737.10
w/osteoporosis	733.0
Osteoporosis	733.00
Otitis Media, Acute	382.9
Chronic	382.9

Fee schedule.

Part III.

A. **Directions:** Use the fee schedule above to complete an encounter form by circling the code and filling in the charges for each patient. Blank encounter forms are on pp. 86-88.

  1. Marilyn Westmoreland, Established patient, Straightforward, Penicillin Injection, Diagnosis Tonsillitis.

  2. Jane Wells, Consultation, High. ECG, Diagnosis Chest pain.

  3. Paula Johnson, New patient, Detailed, Epinephrine Injection, Diagnosis Rash.

Blackburn Primary Care Associates, PC
1990 Turquoise Drive
Blackburn, WI 54937
(608) 459-8857

Howard M. Lawler, MD   11
Joanne R. Hughes, MD   21
Ralph Garcia Lopez, MD   31
TAX ID NO. 00-00000000

GUARANTOR NAME AND ADDRESS	PATIENT NO.	PATIENT NAME	DOCTOR NO.	DATE

	DATE OF BIRTH	TELEPHONE NO.	INSURANCE		
			CODE	DESCRIPTION	CERTIFICATE NO.

OFFICE - NEW

X	CPT	SERVICE	FEE
	99201	Prob Foc/Straight	
	99202	Exp Prob/Straight	
	99203	Detailed/Low	
	99204	Compre/Moderate	
	99205	Compre/High	

OFFICE - ESTABLISHED

X	CPT	SERVICE	FEE
	99211	Nurse/Minimal	
	99212	Prob Foc/Straight	
	99213	Exp Prob/Low	
	99214	Detailed/Moderate	
	99215	Compre/High	

OFFICE - CONSULT

X	CPT	SERVICE	FEE
	99241	Prob/Foc/Straight	
	99242	Exp Prob/Straight	
	99243	Detailed/Low	
	99244	Compre/Moderate	
	99245	Compre/High	

PREVENTIVE CARE - ADULT

X	CPT	SERVICE	FEE
	99385	18-39 Initial	
	99386	40-64 Initial	
	99387	65+ Initial	
	99395	18-39 Periodic	
	99396	40-64 Periodic	
	99397	65+ Periodic	

GASTROENEROLOGY

X	CPT	SERVICE	FEE
	45300	Sigmoidoscopy Rig	
	45305	Sigmoid Rig w/bx	
	45330	Sigmoidoscopy Flex	
	45331	Sigmoid Flex w/bx	
	45378	Colonoscopy Diag	
	45380	Colonoscopy w/bx	
	46600	Anoscopy	

CARDIOLOGY & HEARING

X	CPT	SERVICE	FEE
	93000	EKG (Global)	
	93015	Stress Test (Global)	
	93224	Holter (Global)	
	93225	Holter Hook Up	
	93227	Holter Interpretation	
	94010	Pulm Function Test	
	92551	Audiometry Screen	

INJECTIONS & IMMUNIZATION

X	CPT	SERVICE	FEE
	86585	TB Skin Test	
	90716	Varicella Vaccine	
	90724	Flu Vaccine	
	90732	Pneumovax	
	90718	TD Immunization	
	90782	Injection IM*	
	90788	Injection IM Antibiot*	
		Injection joint*	

REPAIR & DERMATOLOGY

X	CPT	SERVICE	FEE
	17110	Warts: #	
		Tags: #	
		Lesion Excis	
		Lesion Destruct	
	SIZE CM:	SITE:	
	MALIG:	PREMAL/BEN:	
		(Check One Above)	
		Simple Closure	
		Intermed Closure	

OTHER

SUPPLIES/DRUGS*

DRUG NAME:
UNIT/MEASURE:
QUANTITY

SM   MED   MAJOR
(circle one)

FOR ALL INJECTIONS, SUPPLY DRUG
INFORMATION

			SIZE CM:	SITE:	
			10060	I&D Abscess	
			10080	I&D Cyst	

DIAGNOSTIC CODES: ICD-9-CM

☐ 789.0 Abdominal Pain	☐ 782.3 Edema	☐ 614.9 Pelvic Inflammatory Disease	☐ 474.0 Tonsillitis, Chronic
☐ 795.0 Abnormal Pap Smear	☐ 492.8 Emphysema	☐ 685.1 Pilonidal Cyst	☐ 465.9 Upper Respiratory Infection, Acute
☐ 706.1 Acne Vulgaris	☐ V16.0 Family History Of Diabetes	☐ 462 Pharyngitis, Acute	☐ 599.0 Urinary Tract Infection
☐ 477.0 Allergic Rhinitis	☐ 780.6 Fever of Undetermined Origin	☐ 627.1 Postmenopausal Bleeding	☐ V03.9 Vaccination/Bacterial Dis.
☐ 285.9 Anemia, NOS	☐ 578.9 G.I. Bleeding, Unspecified	☐ 625.4 Premenstrual Tension	☐ V06.8 Vaccination/Combination
☐ 281.0 Pernicious	☐ 727.41 Ganglion of Joint	☐ 782.1 Rash	☐ V04.8 Vaccination, Influenza
☐ 411.1 Angina, Unstable	☐ 535.0 Gastritis, Acute	☐ 569.3 Rectal Bleeding	☐ 616.10 Vaginitis, Vulvitis, NOS
☐ 427.9 Arythmia, NOS	☐ V72.3 Arythmia, NOS	☐ 398.90 Rheumatic Heart Disease, NOS	☐ 780.4 Vertigo
☐ 440.9 Arteriosclerosis	☐ 748.0 Headache	☐ 431.9 Sinusitis, Acute, NOS	☐ 787.0 Vomiting, Nausea
☐ 714.0 Arthritis, Rheumatoid	☐ 550.90 Hernia, Inguinal, NOS	☐ 782.1 Skin Eruption, Rash	☐ ___ _____
☐ 414.0 ASHD	☐ 054.9 Herpes Simplex	☐ 845.00 Sprain, Ankle	☐ ___ _____
☐ 493.90 Asthma, Bronchial W/O Status Ast.	☐ 053.9 Herpes Zoster	☐ 848.9 Sprain, Muscle, Unspec. Site	☐ ___ _____
☐ 493.91 Asthma, Bronchial W/Status Ast.	☐ 708.9 Hives/Urticaria	☐ 785.6 Swollen Glands	☐ ___ _____
☐ 466.1 Bronchiolitis, Acute	☐ 401.1 Hypertension, Benign	☐ 246.9 Thyroid Disease, Unspecified	
☐ 466.0 Bronchitis, Acute	☐ 401.0 Hypertension, Malignant	☐ 463 Tonsillitis, Acute	
☐ 727.3 Bursitis	☐ 402.90 Hypertension, W/O CHF		
☐ 786.50 Chest Pain	☐ 244.9 Hypothyroidism, Primary		
☐ 574.20 Cholelithiasis	☐ 380.4 Impacted Cerumen		
☐ 372.30 Conjunctivitis, Unspecified	☐ 487.1 Influenza		
☐ 564.0 Constipation	☐ 564.1 Irritable Bowel Syndrome		
☐ 496 COPD	☐ 464.0 Laryngitis, Acute		
☐ 692.9 Dermatitis, Allergic	☐ 454.9 Leg Varicose Veins		
☐ 250.01 Diabetes Mellitus, ID	☐ 424.0 Mitral Valve Prolapse		
☐ 250.00 Diabetes Mellitus, NID	☐ 412 Myocardial Infarction, Old		
☐ 558.9 Diarrhea	☐ 715.90 Osteoarthritis, Unspec. Site		
☐ 562.11 Diverticulitis	☐ 620.2 Ovarian Cyst		
☐ 562.10 Diverticulosis			

RETURN APPOINTMENT

_____ Days
_____ Weeks
_____ Months

Authorization Number:
▶

BALANCE DUE

DATE OF SERVICE	CPT CODE	DIAGNOSIS CODE(S)	CHARGE

Place of Service:
( ) Office
( ) Emergency Room
( ) Inpatient Hospital
( ) Outpatient Hospital
( ) Nursing Home

TOTAL CHARGE	$
AMOUNT PAID	$
PREVIOUS BAL	$
BALANCE DUE	$

Check #: _____

(Circle Method of Payment)
CASH   CHECK   MC   VISA

Physician's Signature
▶ _____

Encounter form

Blackburn Primary Care Associates, PC
1990 Turquoise Drive
Blackburn, WI 54937
(608) 459-8857

Howard M. Lawler, MD   11
Joanne R. Hughes, MD   21
Ralph Garcia Lopez, MD   31
TAX ID NO. 00-00000000

GUARANTOR NAME AND ADDRESS	PATIENT NO.	PATIENT NAME	DOCTOR NO.	DATE

	DATE OF BIRTH	TELEPHONE NO.	INSURANCE		
			CODE	DESCRIPTION	CERTIFICATE NO.

OFFICE - NEW

X	CPT	SERVICE	FEE
	99201	Prob Foc/Straight	
	99202	Exp Prob/Straight	
	99203	Detailed/Low	
	99204	Compre/Moderate	
	99205	Compre/High	

OFFICE - ESTABLISHED

X	CPT	SERVICE	FEE
	99211	Nurse/Minimal	
	99212	Prob Foc/Straight	
	99213	Exp Prob/Low	
	99214	Detailed/Moderate	
	99215	Compre/High	

OFFICE - CONSULT

X	CPT	SERVICE	FEE
	99241	Prob/Foc/Straight	
	99242	Exp Prob/Straight	
	99243	Detailed/Low	
	99244	Compre/Moderate	
	99245	Compre/High	

PREVENTIVE CARE - ADULT

X	CPT	SERVICE	FEE
	99385	18-39 Initial	
	99386	40-64 Initial	
	99387	65+ Initial	
	99395	18-39 Periodic	
	99396	40-64 Periodic	
	99397	65+ Periodic	

GASTROENEROLOGY

X	CPT	SERVICE	FEE
	45300	Sigmoidoscopy Rig	
	45305	Sigmoid Rig w/bx	
	45330	Sigmoidoscopy Flex	
	45331	Sigmoid Flex w/bx	
	45378	Colonoscopy Diag	
	45380	Colonoscopy w/bx	
	46600	Anoscopy	

CARDIOLOGY & HEARING

X	CPT	SERVICE	FEE
	93000	EKG (Global)	
	93015	Stress Test (Global)	
	93224	Holter (Global)	
	93225	Holter Hook Up	
	93227	Holter Interpretation	
	94010	Pulm Function Test	
	92551	Audiometry Screen	

INJECTIONS & IMMUNIZATION

X	CPT	SERVICE	FEE
	86585	TB Skin Test	
	90716	Varicella Vaccine	
	90724	Flu Vaccine	
	90732	Pneumovax	
	90718	TD Immunization	
	90782	Injection IM*	
	90788	Injection IM Antibiot*	
		Injection joint*	

REPAIR & DERMATOLOGY

X	CPT	SERVICE	FEE
	17110	Warts: #	
		Tags: #	
		Lesion Excis	
		Lesion Destruct	

SIZE CM: SITE:
MALIG: PREMAL/BEN:

(Check One Above)
Simple Closure
Intermed Closure

OTHER

SUPPLIES/DRUGS*

DRUG NAME:
UNIT/MEASURE:
QUANTITY

SM   MED   MAJOR
(circle one)
FOR ALL INJECTIONS, SUPPLY DRUG
INFORMATION

SIZE CM: SITE:

10060	I&D Abscess
10080	I&D Cyst

DIAGNOSTIC CODES: ICD-9-CM

☐ 789.0 Abdominal Pain	☐ 782.3 Edema	☐ 614.9 Pelvic Inflammatory Disease	☐ 474.0 Tonsillitis, Chronic
☐ 795.0 Abnormal Pap Smear	☐ 492.8 Emphysema	☐ 685.1 Pilonidal Cyst	☐ 465.9 Upper Respiratory Infection, Acute
☐ 706.1 Acne Vulgaris	☐ V16.0 Family History Of Diabetes	☐ 462 Pharyngitis, Acute	☐ 599.0 Urinary Tract Infection
☐ 477.0 Allergic Rhinitis	☐ 780.6 Fever of Undetermined Origin	☐ 627.1 Postmenopausal Bleeding	☐ V03.9 Vaccination/Bacterial Dis.
☐ 285.9 Anemia, NOS	☐ 578.9 G.I. Bleeding, Unspecified	☐ 625.4 Premenstrual Tension	☐ V06.8 Vaccination/Combination
☐ 281.0 Pernicious	☐ 727.41 Ganglion of Joint	☐ 782.1 Rash	☐ V04.8 Vaccination, Influenza
☐ 411.1 Angina, Unstable	☐ 535.0 Gastritis, Acute	☐ 569.3 Rectal Bleeding	☐ 616.10 Vaginitis, Vulvitis, NOS
☐ 427.9 Arythmia, NOS	☐ V72.3 Arythmia, NOS	☐ 398.90 Rheumatic Heart Disease, NOS	☐ 780.4 Vertigo
☐ 440.9 Arteriosclerosis	☐ 748.0 Headache	☐ 431.9 Sinusitis, Acute, NOS	☐ 787.0 Vomiting, Nausea
☐ 714.0 Arthritis, Rheumatoid	☐ 550.90 Hernia, Inguinal, NOS	☐ 782.1 Skin Eruption, Rash	☐ ___ ___
☐ 414.0 ASHD	☐ 054.9 Herpes Simplex	☐ 845.00 Sprain, Ankle	☐ ___ ___
☐ 493.90 Asthma, Bronchial W/O Status Ast.	☐ 053.9 Herpes Zoster	☐ 848.9 Sprain, Muscle, Unspec. Site	☐ ___ ___
☐ 493.91 Asthma, Bronchial W/Status Ast.	☐ 708.9 Hives/Urticaria	☐ 785.6 Swollen Glands	☐ ___ ___
☐ 466.1 Bronchiolitis, Acute	☐ 401.1 Hypertension, Benign	☐ 246.9 Thyroid Disease, Unspecified	
☐ 466.0 Bronchitis, Acute	☐ 401.0 Hypertension, Malignant	☐ 463 Tonsillitis, Acute	
☐ 727.3 Bursitis	☐ 402.90 Hypertension, W/O CHF		
☐ 786.50 Chest Pain	☐ 244.9 Hypothyroidism, Primary		
☐ 574.20 Cholelithiasis	☐ 380.4 Impacted Cerumen		
☐ 372.30 Conjunctivitis, Unspecified	☐ 487.1 Influenza		
☐ 564.0 Constipation	☐ 564.1 Irritable Bowel Syndrome		
☐ 496 COPD	☐ 464.0 Laryngitis, Acute		
☐ 692.9 Dermatitis, Allergic	☐ 454.9 Leg Varicose Veins		
☐ 250.01 Diabetes Mellitus, ID	☐ 424.0 Mitral Valve Prolapse		
☐ 250.00 Diabetes Mellitus, NID	☐ 412 Myocardial Infarction, Old		
☐ 558.9 Diarrhea	☐ 715.90 Osteoarthritis, Unspec. Site		
☐ 562.11 Diverticulitis	☐ 620.2 Ovarian Cyst		
☐ 562.10 Diverticulosis			

RETURN APPOINTMENT

_____ Days
_____ Weeks
_____ Months

Authorization Number:
▶ _____

BALANCE DUE

DATE OF SERVICE	CPT CODE	DIAGNOSIS CODE(S)	CHARGE

Place of Service:
( ) Office
( ) Emergency Room
( ) Inpatient Hospital
( ) Outpatient Hospital
( ) Nursing Home

TOTAL CHARGE	$
AMOUNT PAID	$
PREVIOUS BAL	$
BALANCE DUE	$

Check #: _____
(Circle Method of Payment)
CASH   CHECK   MC   VISA

Physician's Signature
▶ _____

Encounter form

Blackburn Primary Care Associates, PC
1990 Turquoise Drive
Blackburn, WI 54937
(608) 459-8857

Howard M. Lawler, MD   11
Joanne R. Hughes, MD   21
Ralph Garcia Lopez, MD   31
TAX ID NO. 00-00000000

GUARANTOR NAME AND ADDRESS	PATIENT NO.	PATIENT NAME	DOCTOR NO.	DATE

	DATE OF BIRTH	TELEPHONE NO.	INSURANCE		
			CODE	DESCRIPTION	CERTIFICATE NO.

OFFICE - NEW

X	CPT	SERVICE	FEE
	99201	Prob Foc/Straight	
	99202	Exp Prob/Straight	
	99203	Detailed/Low	
	99204	Compre/Moderate	
	99205	Compre/High	

OFFICE - ESTABLISHED

X	CPT	SERVICE	FEE
	99211	Nurse/Minimal	
	99212	Prob Foc/Straight	
	99213	Exp Prob/Low	
	99214	Detailed/Moderate	
	99215	Compre/High	

OFFICE - CONSULT

X	CPT	SERVICE	FEE
	99241	Prob/Foc/Straight	
	99242	Exp Prob/Straight	
	99243	Detailed/Low	
	99244	Compre/Moderate	
	99245	Compre/High	

PREVENTIVE CARE - ADULT

X	CPT	SERVICE	FEE
	99385	18-39 Initial	
	99386	40-64 Initial	
	99387	65+ Initial	
	99395	18-39 Periodic	
	99396	40-64 Periodic	
	99397	65+ Periodic	

GASTROENEROLOGY

X	CPT	SERVICE	FEE
	45300	Sigmoidoscopy Rig	
	45305	Sigmoid Rig w/bx	
	45330	Sigmoidoscopy Flex	
	45331	Sigmoid Flex w/bx	
	45378	Colonoscopy Diag	
	45380	Colonoscopy w/bx	
	46600	Anoscopy	

CARDIOLOGY & HEARING

X	CPT	SERVICE	FEE
	93000	EKG (Global)	
	93015	Stress Test (Global)	
	93224	Holter (Global)	
	93225	Holter Hook Up	
	93227	Holter Interpretation	
	94010	Pulm Function Test	
	92551	Audiometry Screen	

INJECTIONS & IMMUNIZATION

X	CPT	SERVICE	FEE
	86585	TB Skin Test	
	90716	Varicella Vaccine	
	90724	Flu Vaccine	
	90732	Pneumovax	
	90718	TD Immunization	
	90782	Injection IM*	
	90788	Injection IM Antibiot*	
		Injection joint*	

REPAIR & DERMATOLOGY

X	CPT	SERVICE	FEE
	17110	Warts: #	
		Tags: #	
		Lesion Excis	
		Lesion Destruct	

SIZE CM: SITE:
MALIG: PREMAL/BEN:

(Check One Above)	
Simple Closure	
Intermed Closure	

SIZE CM: SITE:

OTHER

SUPPLIES/DRUGS*

DRUG NAME:
UNIT/MEASURE:
QUANTITY

SM	MED	MAJOR
(circle one)		

FOR ALL INJECTIONS, SUPPLY DRUG
INFORMATION

	10060	I&D Abscess	
	10080	I&D Cyst	

DIAGNOSTIC CODES: ICD-9-CM

☐ 789.0	Abdominal Pain
☐ 795.0	Abnormal Pap Smear
☐ 706.1	Acne Vulgaris
☐ 477.0	Allergic Rhinitis
☐ 285.9	Anemia, NOS
☐ 281.0	Pernicious
☐ 411.1	Angina, Unstable
☐ 427.9	Arythmia, NOS
☐ 440.9	Arteriosclerosis
☐ 714.0	Arthritis, Rheumatoid
☐ 414.0	ASHD
☐ 493.90	Asthma, Bronchial W/O Status Ast.
☐ 493.91	Asthma, Bronchial W/Status Ast.
☐ 466.1	Bronchiolitis, Acute
☐ 466.0	Bronchitis, Acute
☐ 727.3	Bursitis
☐ 786.50	Chest Pain
☐ 574.20	Cholelithiasis
☐ 372.30	Conjunctivitis, Unspecified
☐ 564.0	Constipation
☐ 496	COPD
☐ 692.9	Dermatitis, Allergic
☐ 250.01	Diabetes Mellitus, ID
☐ 250.00	Diabetes Mellitus, NID
☐ 558.9	Diarrhea
☐ 562.11	Diverticulitis
☐ 562.10	Diverticulosis

☐ 782.3	Edema
☐ 492.8	Emphysema
☐ V16.0	Family History Of Diabetes
☐ 780.6	Fever of Undetermined Origin
☐ 578.9	G.I. Bleeding, Unspecified
☐ 727.41	Ganglion of Joint
☐ 535.0	Gastritis, Acute
☐ V72.3	Arythmia, NOS
☐ 748.0	Headache
☐ 550.90	Hernia, Inguinal, NOS
☐ 054.9	Herpes Simplex
☐ 053.9	Herpes Zoster
☐ 708.9	Hives/Urticaria
☐ 401.1	Hypertension, Benign
☐ 401.0	Hypertension, Malignant
☐ 402.90	Hypertension, W/O CHF
☐ 244.9	Hypothyroidism, Primary
☐ 380.4	Impacted Cerumen
☐ 487.1	Influenza
☐ 564.1	Irritable Bowel Syndrome
☐ 464.0	Laryngitis, Acute
☐ 454.9	Leg Varicose Veins
☐ 424.0	Mitral Valve Prolapse
☐ 412	Myocardial Infarction, Old
☐ 715.90	Osteoarthritis, Unspec. Site
☐ 620.2	Ovarian Cyst

☐ 614.9	Pelvic Inflammatory Disease
☐ 685.1	Pilonidal Cyst
☐ 462	Pharyngitis, Acute
☐ 627.1	Postmenopausal Bleeding
☐ 625.4	Premenstrual Tension
☐ 782.1	Rash
☐ 569.3	Rectal Bleeding
☐ 398.90	Rheumatic Heart Disease, NOS
☐ 431.9	Sinusitis, Acute, NOS
☐ 782.1	Skin Eruption, Rash
☐ 845.00	Sprain, Ankle
☐ 848.9	Sprain, Muscle, Unspec. Site
☐ 785.6	Swollen Glands
☐ 246.9	Thyroid Disease, Unspecified
☐ 463	Tonsillitis, Acute

☐ 474.0	Tonsillitis, Chronic
☐ 465.9	Upper Respiratory Infection, Acute
☐ 599.0	Urinary Tract Infection
☐ V03.9	Vaccination/Bacterial Dis.
☐ V06.8	Vaccination/Combination
☐ V04.8	Vaccination, Influenza
☐ 616.10	Vaginitis, Vulvitis, NOS
☐ 780.4	Vertigo
☐ 787.0	Vomiting, Nausea
☐ ____	_____
☐ ____	_____
☐ ____	_____
☐ ____	_____

RETURN APPOINTMENT

____ Days
____ Weeks
____ Months

Authorization Number:
▶ _____

BALANCE DUE

DATE OF SERVICE	CPT CODE	DIAGNOSIS CODE(S)	CHARGE

Place of Service:
( ) Office
( ) Emergency Room
( ) Inpatient Hospital
( ) Outpatient Hospital
( ) Nursing Home

TOTAL CHARGE	$
AMOUNT PAID	$
PREVIOUS BAL	$
BALANCE DUE	$

Check #: _____
(Circle Method of Payment)
CASH   CHECK   MC   VISA

Physician's Signature
▶ _____

Encounter form

B. **Directions:** Set up a patient ledger for each patient. Refer to p. 113 for an example of a patient ledger. Post the office visit and charges. Record the following payments and balances on the sample page provided below.

1. Marilyn Westmoreland paid $10 copayment.

2. Jane Wells paid $75.

3. Paula Johnson paid bill in full.

C. Post all three transactions in the daily journal.

JOURNAL OF DAILY CHARGES, PAYMENTS & DEPOSITS

PLACE FIRST PEG HERE

	DATE	PROFESSIONAL SERVICE	FEE	PAYMENT	ADJUST-MENT	NEW BALANCE	OLD BALANCE	PATIENT'S NAME	
1									1
2									2
3									3
4									4
5									5
6									6
7									7
8									8
9									9
10									10
11									11
12									12
13									13
14									14
15									15
16									16
17									17
18									18
19									19
20									20
21									21
22									22
23									23
24									24
25									25
26									26
27									27
28									28
29									29
30									30
31								TOTALS THIS PAGE	31
32								TOTALS PREVIOUS PAGE	32
33								TOTALS MONTH TO DATE	33

COLUMN A   COLUMN B   COLUMN C   COLUMN D   COLUMN E

MEMO _____

_____

_____

_____

DAILY-FROM LINE 31

ARITHMETIC POSTING PROOF	
Column E	
Plus Column A	
Sub-Total	
Minus Column B	
Sub-Total	
Minus Column C	
Equals Column D	

Box 1

MONTH-FROM LINE 31

ARITHMETIC POSTING PROOF	
Accts. Receivable Previous Day	$
Plus Column A	
Sub-Total	
Minus Column B	
Sub-Total	
Minus Column C	
Accts. Receivable End of Day	

Box 2

Daily journal

Part IV.

A. **Directions:** Complete the following statements.

1. When a statement is returned marked "Moved—no forwarding address," you may consider this account as a _____.

2. A telephone call at the right time, in the right manner, is more effective than a

_____.

3. Collection by an agency will mean sacrificing from _____ to _____ of the amount owed.

B. **Directions:** List six guidelines for handling an account that has been turned over to collections.

1. _____
2. _____
3. _____
4. _____
5. _____
6. _____

C. **Directions:** Describe the following.

1. Fair Debt Collection Practices Act

_____

2. Regulation Z of the Truth in Lending Act

_____

3. Small Claims Court

_____

D. **Directions:** Discuss with a classmate how you feel about making collection calls or asking for payment. Rehearse various ways to ask for payment.

_____
_____
_____
_____
_____
_____
_____
_____

CHAPTER 15

Basics of Diagnostic Coding

Part I.

Symbols, abbreviations, punctuation, and notations appear in the listings to serve as instructional notes. Understanding their meaning and using them for guidance are crucial to accurate coding.

Directions: Fill in the blanks with the appropriate vocabulary terms.

1. □ The _____ symbol precedes a disease code to indicate that the content of a four-digit category has been moved or modified.

2. § This _____ _____ symbol is only used in the Tabular List of Diseases.

3. ● The _____ symbol indicates a new entry.

4. ▲ The _____ indicates a revision in the Tabular List of Diseases and a code change in the alphabetical index.

5. ▶◀ These symbols mark both the _____ and _____ of new or revised text.

6. ♀ _____ diagnosis only.

7. ♂ _____ diagnosis only.

8. √4th Code requires a _____ digit.

9. √5th Code requires a _____ digit.

10. [ ] _____ are used to enclose synonyms, alternative wordings, or explanatory phrases.

11. ( ) _____ are used to enclose supplementary words, which may be present or absent in the statement of a disease or procedure without affecting the code number to which it is assigned.

12. : A _____ is used in the Tabular List of Diseases after an incomplete term that needs one or more of the modifiers that follow it to make the assignable to a given category.

13. {} _____ enclose a series of terms, each of which is modified by the statement appearing to the right of the brace.

Part II. _____

Directions: Using this checklist, code the diagnoses listed below.

- Identify the key terms in the diagnostic statement, determining the main reason for the encounter.

- Locate the diagnosis in the alphabetic index (volume II).

- Read and understand any footnotes, symbols, or instructions following any cross-references.

- Locate the diagnosis in the Tabular List of Diseases.

- Read and understand the inclusions and exclusions.

- Make sure you include fourth and fifth digits when available, assigning to the highest level of specificity.

- Assign the code, until all diagnosis elements are identified.

- After assigning the code, double-check to ensure accurate transfer from the book to the patient form and subsequent data entry.

- Use the same process for secondary diagnoses and other conditions addressed during the encounter.

Diagnosis	International Classification of Diseases, Ninth Revision (ICD-9) Code
1. Polycystic kidney	
2. Amenorrhea	
3. Measles	
4. Hematuria	
5. Catatonic schizophrenia, chronic	
6. Cancer of the duodenum (neoplasm)	
7. Nodular tuberculosis (lung)	
8. High blood pressure	
9. Left-sided congestive heart failure	
10. Croup	
11. Ear wax	
12. Exophthalmos R/T thyroid	
13. Gout	
14. Active rickets	
15. Cat scratch fever	
16. Benign prostatic hypertrophy (enlarged prostate)	
17. Encephalitis from West Nile virus	
18. Thrush	
19. Parkinson's disease	

Diagnosis	International Classification of Diseases, Ninth Revision *(ICD-9)* Code
20. Senile cataract	
21. Huntington's chorea	
22. Mitral valve prolapse	
23. Transient ischemic attack	
24. Asthma	
25. Cushing's syndrome	

Diagnosis	V-Code
1. Ear piercing	
2. Gynecologic exam	
3. Annual physical	
4. Venereal disease exposure	
5. History of mental illness	

Situation	E-Code
1. Bathtub drowning	
2. Rattlesnake bite	
3. Sunstroke	
4. Pedestrian hit by a train	
5. Parachute failure	

Part III.

A. **Directions:** Fill in the blanks.

1. Volume I contains _____ appendices and _____ chapters.

2. _____ is referred to as the *Tabular List of Diseases*.

3. Volume II contains an _____ index of disease and injury.

B. **Directions:** Complete Box 21 of the Health Care Financing Administration (HCFA) 1500 form by writing in the *International Classification of Diseases, Ninth Revision (ICD-9)* codes that you found for Part II.

1. Gout and hypertension (code as primary)

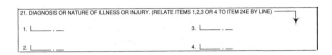

2. Croup and thrush

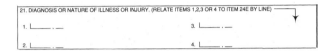

3. Hematuria and benign prostatic hypertrophy (code as primary)

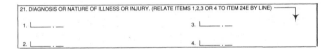

4. Left-sided congestive heart failure and gout

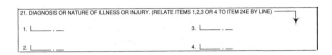

Part IV.

A. Why would an *ICD-9* coding book be a good reference tool for a medical transcriptionist?

_____

_____

_____

_____

B. Indicate which statements are true (T) and which statements are false (F).

1. _____ Documentation regarding preexisting condition is required.

2. _____ Conditions described as "rule out," "suspected," "probable," or "questionable" should be coded.

3. _____ It is okay to substitute another *ICD-9* code if a patient requests that a diagnosis other than the correct or appropriate diagnosis be used for the visit because that patient's insurance company will not reimburse for the actual diagnosis.

4. _____ You have a legal and ethical responsibility to code the diagnosis correctly.

5. _____ If no definitive diagnosis is made, the symptoms should be coded.

CHAPTER 16

Basics of Procedural Coding

Part I. Vocabulary

Directions: Fill in the blanks with the appropriate vocabulary terms.

A. *Current Procedural Terminology (CPT)* was first published in _____ by the American Medical Association (AMA). It was based on the California Relative Value Study, developed by the California Medical Society. Its primary purpose was to simplify the reporting of

_____ and/or _____ provided by physicians.

B. 1992 marked the most significant change to *CPT,* with the replacement of the office and hospital

visit codes with the _____ (E&M) codes, identifying key elements to be documented in the medical record.

C. *CPT* has been revised three times, and the edition in current use is _____.

D. *CPT* is updated every _____ by the AMA and published for the next calendar year.

E. _____ codes describe procedures or services that are grouped together and paid as one. An example would be code 90700 for a Diphtheria, Tetanus, and Pertussis vaccine for intramuscular use.

F. _____ codes means reporting the components of a procedure separately. In the example above (code 90700), if you report the three vaccines separately, it gives the impression that three injections, and not one, were given.

G. _____ is a deliberate increase in a *CPT* code to receive higher reimbursements. This is a target of Centers for Medicare & Medicaid Services (CMS) investigations and should never be done.

H. _____ is usually done by insurance companies for several reasons, either when one coding system is converted to another or if, on review, the examiner believes the documentation does not match the code description.

Part II.

Directions: Use these steps in *CPT* coding to find the following codes.

- Know your *CPT* code book: changes are made each year, so even if you have been coding for years, you need to read the introduction, guidelines, and notes.

- Review all services and procedures performed on the day of the encounter; include all medications administered and trays and equipment used.

- Find the procedures and/or services in the index in the back of the *CPT* book. This will direct you to a code (not a page number). The code you are looking for may be listed as a procedure, body system, service, or abbreviation (which will usually refer you to the full spelling).

- Read the description in the code and also any related descriptions that follow a semicolon; this will lead you to the most accurate code.

- If the service is an Evaluation and Management code do the following:

  Determine whether the person is a new or established patient.

  Determine whether this is a consultation.

  Indicate where the service was performed.

  Review the documentation to determine the level of service.

  Check to see whether there is a reason to use a modifier.

  Assign the five-digit *CPT* code.

Procedure	*CPT* Code
1. Liver biopsy, needle	
2. Cholecystectomy	
3. Newborn circumcision	
4. Gastric motility study	
5. Right heart catheterization	
6. Intradermal allergy testing	
7. Removal of foreign body from nose	
8. X-ray examination of ankle, three views	
9. Computed axial tomography (CAT) scan of arm with contrast	
10. Partial thromboplastin time (PTT)	

Find the Appropriate Modifier	Modifier
1. Bilateral	
2. Two surgeons	
3. Repeat procedure same surgeon	
4. Multiple procedures	

Part III.

A. Symbols appear in the listings to serve as instructional notes. Understanding their meaning and using them for guidance are crucial to accurate coding.

Directions: Describe each symbol.

1. ● _____ procedure

2. ▲ code _____

3. + *CPT* _____ codes

4. Ø exempt from the use of _____ –51

5. ▶◀ revised _____, cross-_____ and explanations

6. → with a circle around it, which refers to *CPT* _____

7. * _____ procedure only

B. **Directions:** Look at a *CPT* book and list the sections.

1. _____

2. _____

3. _____

4. _____

5. _____

Part IV. _____

A. What three things must you know before assigning an E&M code?

1. _____

2. _____

3. _____

B. Name the four levels of histories.

1. _____

2. _____

3. _____

4. _____

C. List the four levels of decision making.

1. _____

2. _____

3. _____

4. _____

D. Insert the appropriate E&M code in Box 24 of the Health Care Financing Administration (HCFA) 1500 form and relate it to the matching diagnosis in Box 21. Indicate the relationship in column E of Box 24.

1. New patient, comprehensive exam and history, 45 minutes, *International Classification of Diseases, Ninth Revision (ICD-9)* code for physical exam V70.0 and use 11 (doctor's office) for place of service in column B.

```
21. DIAGNOSIS OR NATURE OF ILLNESS OR INJURY. (RELATE ITEMS 1,2,3 OR 4 TO ITEM 24E BY LINE)
1. L___ . __              3. L___ . __
2. L___ . __              4. L___ . __
```

24.	A						B	C	D		E	F	G	H	I	J	K
	DATE(S) OF SERVICE						Place of Service	Type of Service	PROCEDURES, SERVICES, OR SUPPLIES (Explain Unusual Circumstances)		DIAGNOSIS CODE	$ CHARGES	DAYS OR UNITS	EPSDT Family Plan	EMG	COB	RESERVED FOR LOCAL USE
	From			To					CPT/HCPCS	MODIFIER							
	MM	DD	YY	MM	DD	YY											
1																	
2																	
3																	
4																	
5																	
6																	

2. Established patient, problem-focused exam and history, 10 minutes, *ICD-9* code for anemia is 281.9 and use 11 (doctor's office) for place of service in column B.

21. DIAGNOSIS OR NATURE OF ILLNESS OR INJURY. (RELATE ITEMS 1,2,3 OR 4 TO ITEM 24E BY LINE)

1. └___.__   3. └___.__

2. └___.__   4. └___.__

24.	A						B	C	D		E	F	G	H	I	J	K
	DATE(S) OF SERVICE						Place of Service	Type of Service	PROCEDURES, SERVICES, OR SUPPLIES (Explain Unusual Circumstances)		DIAGNOSIS CODE	$ CHARGES	DAYS OR UNITS	EPSDT Family Plan	EMG	COB	RESERVED FOR LOCAL USE
	From			To					CPT/HCPCS	MODIFIER							
	MM	DD	YY	MM	DD	YY											
1																	
2																	
3																	
4																	
5																	
6																	

3. Established patient, detailed exam and history, 25 minutes, *ICD-9* code for cervical cancer is 180.9. She also has anxiety, which is a secondary diagnosis of 308.3. A Papanicolaou smear *CPT* 88141 is performed. Use 11 (doctor's office) for place of service in column B.

21. DIAGNOSIS OR NATURE OF ILLNESS OR INJURY. (RELATE ITEMS 1,2,3 OR 4 TO ITEM 24E BY LINE)

1. └___.__   3. └___.__

2. └___.__   4. └___.__

24.	A						B	C	D		E	F	G	H	I	J	K
	DATE(S) OF SERVICE						Place of Service	Type of Service	PROCEDURES, SERVICES, OR SUPPLIES (Explain Unusual Circumstances)		DIAGNOSIS CODE	$ CHARGES	DAYS OR UNITS	EPSDT Family Plan	EMG	COB	RESERVED FOR LOCAL USE
	From			To					CPT/HCPCS	MODIFIER							
	MM	DD	YY	MM	DD	YY											
1																	
2																	
3																	
4																	
5																	
6																	

CHAPTER 17

The Health Insurance Claim Form

Part I. _____

List some of the advantages and disadvantages of paper claims.

1. _____

2. _____

3. _____

4. _____

List some of the advantages and disadvantages of electronic claims.

1. _____

2. _____

3. _____

4. _____

Part II. _____

A. **Directions:** Use the information included in this chapter to complete a registration form for a patient who was referred by Dr. Mills.

REGISTRATION
(PLEASE PRINT)

Home Phone: _____   Today's Date: _____

PATIENT INFORMATION

Name_____   Soc. Sec.# _____
           Last Name   First Name   Initial

Address_____

City _____ State _____ Zip _____

Single ___ Married ___ Widowed ___ Separated ___ Divorced ___ Sex M___ F___ Age ___ Birthdate _____

Patient Employed by _____ Occupation _____

Business Address _____ Business Phone _____

By whom were you referred? _____

In case of emergency who should be notified? _____ Phone _____
                                              Last Name   Relationship to Patient

PRIMARY INSURANCE

Person Responsible for Account _____
                                    Last Name   First Name   Initial

Relation to Patient _____ Birthdate _____ Soc. Sec.# _____

Address (if different from patient's) _____ Phone _____

City _____ State _____ Zip _____

Person Responsible Employed by _____ Occupation _____

Business Address _____ Business Phone _____

Insurance Company_____

Contract # _____ Group # _____ Subscriber # _____

Name of other dependents covered under this plan _____

ADDITIONAL INSURANCE

Is patient covered by additional insurance?   ____ Yes ____ No

Subscriber Name _____ Relationship to Patient _____ Birthdate _____

Address (if different from patient's) _____ Phone _____

City _____ State _____ Zip _____

Subscriber Employed by _____ Business Phone _____

Insurance Company _____

Contract # _____ Group # _____ Subscriber # _____

Name of other dependents covered under this plan _____

ASSIGNMENT AND RELEASE

I, the undersigned, certify that I (or my dependent) have insurance coverage with _____
                                                                                  Name of Insurance Company(ies)
and assign directly to Dr. _____ insurance benefits, if any, otherwise payable to me for services rendered. I
understand that I am financially responsible for all charges whether or not paid by insurance. I hereby authorize the doctor to release
all information necessary to secure the payment of benefits. I authorize the use of this signature on all insurance submissions.

_____   _____   _____
  Responsible Party Signature   Relationship   Date

ORDER# 58-8426 • © 1996 BIBBERO SYSTEMS, INC. • PETALUMA, CALIFORNIA • TO REORDER CALL TOLL FREE: (800) 242-9330

Sample registration form.

B. **Directions:** Complete as many boxes as you can by using the following information. Indicate who may sign the various signature boxes.

John M. Smith, Father, DOB 10-25-67 ID#123456789 Mary L. Smith, Mother, DOB 9-29-69 ID#987654321 Levi Smith, Patient, DOB 9-11-96, male	Blackburn Realty (Acme Insurance Group #12345) Diamonte Hospital (BCBS Insurance Group #5432) Child (student) Blackburn Middle School Child is insured by both parents. Mom's insurance is primary because of her birth month.
Date of Illness 4-15-20XX Similar illness last month 3-12-20XX Diagnosis Croup 464.4 Office Visit Established Patient, 15 min 99213, $86 Referred by Dr. Fred Mills ID#123-6543-8761	Patient Address: 408 West View Road Blackburn, IL 123456 (123) 555-5432

1. MEDICARE	MEDICAID	CHAMPUS	CHAMPVA	GROUP HEALTH PLAN	FECA BLK LUNG	OTHER
☐ (Medicare #)	☐ (Medicaid #)	☐ (Sponsor's SSN)	☐ (VA File #)	☐ (SSN or ID)	☐ (SSN)•	☐ (ID)

1a. INSURED'S I.D. NUMBER   (FOR PROGRAM IN ITEM 1)

2. PATIENT'S NAME (Last Name, First Name, Middle Initial)

3. PATIENT'S BIRTH DATE
MM   DD   YY   SEX
                M ☐   F ☐

4. INSURED'S NAME (Last Name, First Name, Middle Initial)

5. PATIENT'S ADDRESS (No., Street)

CITY   STATE

ZIP CODE   TELEPHONE (Include Area Code)
                  (   )

6. PATIENT RELATIONSHIP TO INSURED
Self ☐   Spouse ☐   Child ☐   Other ☐

7. INSURED'S ADDRESS (No., Street)

CITY   STATE

ZIP CODE   TELEPHONE (INCLUDE AREA CODE)
                  (   )

8. PATIENT STATUS
Single ☐   Married ☐   Other ☐

Employed ☐   Full-Time Student ☐   Part-Time Student ☐

9. OTHER INSURED'S NAME (Last Name, First Name, Middle Initial)

a. OTHER INSURED'S POLICY OR GROUP NUMBER

b. OTHER INSURED'S DATE OF BIRTH   SEX
MM   DD   YY
M ☐   F ☐

c. EMPLOYER'S NAME OR SCHOOL NAME

d. INSURANCE PLAN NAME OR PROGRAM NAME

10. IS PATIENT'S CONDITION RELATED TO:

a. EMPLOYMENT? (CURRENT OR PREVIOUS)
☐ YES   ☐ NO

b. AUTO ACCIDENT?   PLACE (State)
☐ YES   ☐ NO   └___┘

c. OTHER ACCIDENT?
☐ YES   ☐ NO

11. INSURED'S POLICY GROUP OR FECA NUMBER

a. INSURED'S DATE OF BIRTH   SEX
MM   DD   YY
M ☐   F ☐

b. EMPLOYER'S NAME OR SCHOOL NAME

c. INSURANCE PLAN NAME OR PROGRAM NAME

d. IS THERE ANOTHER HEALTH BENEFIT PLAN?
☐ YES   ☐ NO   **If yes**, return to and complete item 9 a-d.

READ BACK OF FORM BEFORE COMPLETING & SIGNING THIS FORM.
12. PATIENT'S OR AUTHORIZED PERSON'S SIGNATURE I authorize the release of any medical or other information necessary to process this claim. I also request payment of government benefits either to myself or to the party who accepts assignment below.

SIGNED _____   DATE _____

13. INSURED'S OR AUTHORIZED PERSON'S SIGNATURE I authorize payment of medical benefits to the undersigned physician or supplier for services described below.

SIGNED _____

14. DATE OF CURRENT: ◀ ILLNESS (First symptom) OR
MM   DD   YY   INJURY (Accident) OR
    PREGNANCY(LMP)

15. IF PATIENT HAS HAD SAME OR SIMILAR ILLNESS.
GIVE FIRST DATE   MM   DD   YY

16. DATES PATIENT UNABLE TO WORK IN CURRENT OCCUPATION
    MM   DD   YY   MM   DD   YY
FROM   TO

17. NAME OF REFERRING PHYSICIAN OR OTHER SOURCE

17a. I.D. NUMBER OF REFERRING PHYSICIAN

21. DIAGNOSIS OR NATURE OF ILLNESS OR INJURY. (RELATE ITEMS 1,2,3 OR 4 TO ITEM 24E BY LINE) ┐
                                             ▼

1. └___. ___   3. └___. ___

2. └___. ___   4. └___. ___

24.	A DATE(S) OF SERVICE			To			B Place of Service	C Type of Service	D PROCEDURES, SERVICES, OR SUPPLIES (Explain Unusual Circumstances)		E DIAGNOSIS CODE	F $ CHARGES	G DAYS OR UNITS	H EPSDT Family Plan	I EMG	J COB	K RESERVED FOR LOCAL USE
	From MM	DD	YY	MM	DD	YY			CPT/HCPCS	MODIFIER							
1																	
2																	
3																	
4																	
5																	
6																	

Part III.

Directions: Use the insurance log to answer the following questions.

1. For how many visits was Terry Holmes charged? _____

2. How much did the patient pay on the second visit? _____

3. How much did insurance pay for the first visit? _____

4. What was the patient's balance after insurance paid for the second visit? _____

5. How much did insurance pay for the last visit? _____

6. What does the patient need to be reimbursed? _____

General Physicians, Inc.
5515 Lake Dr.
Chicago, IL 00000

INSURANCE LOG

Patient's Name	Date of Service	Fee	Amt. Paid	Insurance Reimbursements		Amt. Due from Patient	Date	Amt. Reimbursed to Patient	Date	Current Balance
				Date	Amount					
Terry Holmes	2/5/03	$85	0	3/15/03	$75	$10	3/15			
	2/17/03	$30	30	3/30/03	$25	$5	3/30			
	3/24/03	$65	40	4/15/03	$32			$22	5/25/03	0

Insurance log.

Part IV.

Complete a Health Care Financing Administration (HCFA) 1500 form below for yourself using your own address and insurance information. Use Diagnosis V70.0, E&M Code 99213, and $65 for charges.

PLEASE
DO NOT
STAPLE
IN THIS
AREA

	PICA		HEALTH INSURANCE CLAIM FORM	PICA	

CARRIER

1. MEDICARE MEDICAID CHAMPUS CHAMPVA GROUP HEALTH PLAN FECA BLK LUNG OTHER	1a. INSURED'S I.D. NUMBER (FOR PROGRAM IN ITEM 1)
(Medicare #) (Medicaid #) (SponsorÕs SSN) (VA File #) (SSN or ID) (SN) (ID)	

2. PATIENT'S NAME (Last Name, First Name, Middle Initial)	3. PATIENT'S BIRTH DATE MM ¦ DD ¦ YY SEX M F	4. INSURED'S NAME (Last Name, First Name, Middle Initial)

5. PATIENT'S ADDRESS (No., Street)	6. PATIENT RELATIONSHIP TO INSURED Self Spouse Child Other	7. INSURED'S ADDRESS (No., Street)

CITY	STATE	8. PATIENT STATUS Single Married Other	CITY	STATE

ZIP CODE	TELEPHONE (Include Area Code) ( )	Employed Full-Time Student Part-Time Student	ZIP CODE	TELEPHONE (INCLUDE AREA CODE) ( )

9. OTHER INSURED'S NAME (Last Name, First Name, Middle Initial)	10. IS PATIENT'S CONDITION RELATED TO:	11. INSURED'S POLICY GROUP OR FECA NUMBER

a. OTHER INSURED'S POLICY OR GROUP NUMBER	a. EMPLOYMENT? (CURRENT OR PREVIOUS) YES NO	a. INSURED'S DATE OF BIRTH MM ¦ DD ¦ YY SEX M F

b. OTHER INSURED'S DATE OF BIRTH MM ¦ DD ¦ YY SEX M F	b. AUTO ACCIDENT? PLACE (State) YES NO	b. EMPLOYER'S NAME OR SCHOOL NAME

c. EMPLOYER'S NAME OR SCHOOL NAME	c. OTHER ACCIDENT? YES NO	c. INSURANCE PLAN NAME OR PROGRAM NAME

d. INSURANCE PLAN NAME OR PROGRAM NAME	10d. RESERVED FOR LOCAL USE	d. IS THERE ANOTHER HEALTH BENEFIT PLAN? YES NO *If yes,* return to and complete item 9 a-d.

PATIENT AND INSURED INFORMATION

READ BACK OF FORM BEFORE COMPLETING & SIGNING THIS FORM. 12. PATIENT'S OR AUTHORIZED PERSON'S SIGNATURE I authorize the release of any medical or other information necessary to process this claim. I also request payment of government benefits either to myself or to the party who accepts assignment below. SIGNED _____ DATE _____	13. INSURED'S OR AUTHORIZED PERSON'S SIGNATURE I authorize payment of medical benefits to the undersigned physician or supplier for services described below. SIGNED _____

14. DATE OF CURRENT: MM ¦ DD ¦ YY ILLNESS (First symptom) OR INJURY (Accident) OR PREGNANCY(LMP)	15. IF PATIENT HAS HAD SAME OR SIMILAR ILLNESS. GIVE FIRST DATE MM ¦ DD ¦ YY	16. DATES PATIENT UNABLE TO WORK IN CURRENT OCCUPATION MM ¦ DD ¦ YY MM ¦ DD ¦ YY FROM TO

17. NAME OF REFERRING PHYSICIAN OR OTHER SOURCE	17a. I.D. NUMBER OF REFERRING PHYSICIAN	18. HOSPITALIZATION DATES RELATED TO CURRENT SERVICES MM ¦ DD ¦ YY MM ¦ DD ¦ YY FROM TO

19. RESERVED FOR LOCAL USE	20. OUTSIDE LAB? YES NO $ CHARGES

21. DIAGNOSIS OR NATURE OF ILLNESS OR INJURY. (RELATE ITEMS 1,2,3 OR 4 TO ITEM 24E BY LINE) 1. L___ . __ 3. L___ . __ 2. L___ . __ 4. L___ . __	22. MEDICAID RESUBMISSION CODE ORIGINAL REF. NO.
	23. PRIOR AUTHORIZATION NUMBER

24. A DATE(S) OF SERVICE From To MM DD YY MM DD YY	B Place of Service	C Type of Service	D PROCEDURES, SERVICES, OR SUPPLIES (Explain Unusual Circumstances) CPT/HCPCS ¦ MODIFIER	E DIAGNOSIS CODE	F $ CHARGES	G DAYS OR UNITS	H EPSDT Family Plan	I EMG	J COB	K RESERVED FOR LOCAL USE
1										
2										
3										
4										
5										
6										

25. FEDERAL TAX I.D. NUMBER SSN EIN	26. PATIENT'S ACCOUNT NO.	27. ACCEPT ASSIGNMENT? (For govt. claims, see back) YES NO	28. TOTAL CHARGE $	29. AMOUNT PAID $	30. BALANCE DUE $

31. SIGNATURE OF PHYSICIAN OR SUPPLIER INCLUDING DEGREES OR CREDENTIALS (I certify that the statements on the reverse apply to this bill and are made a part thereof.) SIGNED _____ DATE _____	32. NAME AND ADDRESS OF FACILITY WHERE SERVICES WERE RENDERED (If other than home or office)	33. PHYSICIAN'S, SUPPLIER'S BILLING NAME, ADDRESS, ZIP CODE & PHONE # PIN# GRP#

PHYSICIAN OR SUPPLIER INFORMATION

(APPROVED BY AMA COUNCIL ON MEDICAL SERVICE 8/88)   ***PLEASE PRINT OR TYPE***   APPROVED OMB-0938-0008 FORM CMS-1500 (12-90),   FORM RRB-1500,
APPROVED OMB-1215-0055 FORM OWCP-1500,   APPROVED OMB-0720-0001 (CHAMPUS)

CHAPTER 18

Third-Party Reimbursement

Part I.

Directions: Define the following insurance terms in your own words.

1. allowed charge

_____

_____

_____

2. authorization

_____

_____

_____

3. benefits

_____

_____

_____

4. birthday rule

_____

_____

_____

5. coordination of benefits

_____

_____

_____

6. copayment

_____

_____

_____

7. deductible

_____

_____

_____

8. government plan

_____

_____

_____

9. group policy

_____

_____

_____

10. health insurance

_____

_____

_____

11. HMO

_____

_____

_____

12. indemnity plan

_____

_____

_____

13. individual policy

_____

_____

_____

14. managed care

_____

_____

_____

15. medical savings account

_____

_____

_____

16. medically indigent

_____

_____

_____

17. medically necessary

_____

_____

_____

18. participating provider

_____

_____

_____

19. policyholder

_____

_____

_____

20. primary diagnosis

_____

_____

_____

21. principal diagnosis

_____

_____

_____

22. premium

_____

_____

_____

23. RBRVS

_____

_____

_____

24. rider

_____

_____

_____

25. self-insured plans

_____

_____

_____

26. service benefit plan

_____

_____

_____

27. workers' compensation

_____

_____

_____

28. utilization review

_____

_____

_____

Part II. _____

A. Name five different types of health insurance plans.

1. _____

2. _____

3. _____

4. _____

5. _____

B. Name seven different types of insurance benefits.

1. _____

2. _____

3. _____

4. _____

5. _____

6. _____

7. _____

Part III. _____

A. List the advantages of managed care.

1. _____

2. _____

3. _____

4. _____

5. _____

B. List the disadvantages of managed care.

1. _____

2. _____

3. _____

4. _____

5. _____

Part IV. _____

Discussion Questions

Directions: Answer the following questions. Be prepared to discuss your answers with your classmates.

1. What is the difference between Medicare and Medicaid?

_____

_____

_____

_____

_____

2. How do CHAMPUS, CHAMPVA, and TRICARE differ?

_____

_____

_____

_____

3. What is the difference between Medicare Part A and Medicare Part B?

_____

_____

_____

_____

4. What is the difference between an HMO and a PPO?

_____

_____

_____

_____

5. What is workers' compensation?

_____

_____

_____

_____

CHAPTER 19

Banking Services and Procedures

Part I. Vocabulary

Directions: Match the following terms and definitions.

1. _____ The process of proving that the blank statement and the checkbook balance are in agreement.

2. _____ Networks of banks that exchange checks with each other.

3. _____ The person presenting the check for payment.

4. _____ Bank or facility from which the check is drawn or written.

5. _____ The person who wrote the check.

6. _____ Electronic banking via computer modem or over the Internet.

7. _____ Person who signs his or her name on the back of a check for the purpose of transferring payment to another person.

8. _____ Money (funds) paid out.

9. _____ Banking through the use of wireless devices, such as cellular phones and wireless Internet services.

10. _____ Any individual, corporation, or legal party who signs a check or any type of negotiable instrument.

11. _____ Legally transferable to another party.

12. _____ Person named on a draft or check as the recipient of the amount shown.

13. _____ Person who writes a check in favor of the payee.

14. _____ A legal statement in which a person authorizes another person to act as his or her attorney or agent. The authority may be limited to the handling of specific procedures. The person authorized to act as the agent is known as *the attorney in fact*.

15. _____ A capital sum of money due as a debt or used as a fund for which interest is either charged or paid.

A. drawee

B. bank reconciliation

C. principal

D. payee

E. negotiable

F. M-banking

G. drawer

H. endorser

I. disbursements

J. holder

K. maker (of a check)

L. e-banking

M. power of attorney

N. payer

O. clearinghouses

Part II.

A. List and describe seven types of checks.

1. _____

2. _____

3. _____

4. _____

5. _____

6. _____

7. _____

B. On the patient ledger on p. 113, record the following transactions.

1. Previous balance $267.00.

2. Office visit 6-1-20XX $76.00.

3. Copayment, $10 received by check #2365 from patient on 6-1-20XX.

4. Insurance payment received $55.00 on 6-13-XX.

5. From the EOB, post an insurance adjustment of $11.00. You are a member of their network.

6. On 6-14-20XX, you received the patient's check returned from the bank for nonsufficient funds. Adjust the account.

7. Add a $10.00 returned check charge, per office policy.

8. What is the patient's balance? _____

Name _____

Date _____

Grade _____

PATIENT LEDGER

BLACKBURN PRIMARY CARE ASSOCIATES, PC
1990 Turquiose Drive
Blackburn, WI 54937
608-459-8857

STATEMENT TO:

				PREVIOUS BALANCE	
DATE	PROFESSIONAL SERVICE	CHARGE	PAYMENT	ADJUST-MENT	NEW BALANCE

Sample patient ledger.

C. Describe each type of endorsement.

1. Blank _____

2. Restrictive _____

3. Special _____

4. Qualified _____

D. Describe two ways a medical assistant can endorse a check.

1. _____

2. _____

E. List five reasons that checks should be deposited promptly.

1. _____

2. _____

3. _____

4. _____

5. _____

Part III. _____

A. What is the ABA number on the checks below? _____

B. What is the account number? _____

C. What are the check numbers? _____

1837			BLACKBURN PRIMARY CARE ASSOCIATES, PC	1837

DATE _____
TO _____
FOR _____

BALANCE BROUGHT FORWARD		
DEPOSITS		
BALANCE		
AMT THIS CK		
BALANCE CARRIED FORWARD		

BLACKBURN PRIMARY CARE ASSOCIATES, PC
1990 Turquoise Drive
Blackburn, WI 54937
608-459-8857

94-72/1224

DATE

PAY TO THE ORDER OF _____ $ [   ]

_____ DOLLARS

DERBYSHIRE SAVINGS Member FDIC
P.O. BOX 8923
Blackburn, WI 54937

FOR

⑈055003⑈ 446782011⑈ 678800470

1838

DATE _____
TO _____
FOR _____

BALANCE BROUGHT FORWARD		
DEPOSITS		
BALANCE		
AMT THIS CK		
BALANCE CARRIED FORWARD		

BLACKBURN PRIMARY CARE ASSOCIATES, PC
1990 Turquoise Drive
Blackburn, WI 54937
608-459-8857

1838

94-72/1224

DATE

PAY TO THE ORDER OF _____ $ [   ]

_____ DOLLARS

DERBYSHIRE SAVINGS Member FDIC
P.O. BOX 8923
Blackburn, WI 54937

FOR

⑈055003⑈ 446782011⑈ 678800470

Sample checks

1839

DATE _____
TO _____
FOR _____

BALANCE BROUGHT FORWARD		
DEPOSITS		
BALANCE		
AMT THIS CK		
BALANCE CARRIED FORWARD		

BLACKBURN PRIMARY CARE ASSOCIATES, PC
1990 Turquoise Drive
Blackburn, WI 54937
608-459-8857

1839

94-72/1224

DATE _____

PAY TO THE
ORDER OF _____ $ [ ]

_____ _DOLLARS_

DERBYSHIRE SAVINGS Member FDIC
P.O. BOX 8923
Blackburn, WI 54937

FOR _____

⑈055003⑈ 446782011⑈ 678800470

SAMPLE

Sample checks—cont'd.

D. Write a check to American Medical Association for $356.00 for coding books (supplies). The beginning balance was $4562.79.

E. Pay the water bill to Blackburn Utility Company for $39.83.

F. Write a check for the office rent to Turquoise Drive Realty for $1700.00. Indicate a deposit of $2230.00.

G. Record these three payments in the disbursement journal.

Name _____
Date _____
Grade _____

DISBURSEMENT RECORD

Check No.	Name	Date	Amount	Deposit	Beg.Balance / Balance	1 Supplies	2 Salary	3 Rent	4 Misc.

Sample disbursement record.

H. Prepare a bank deposit detail for the $2230.00 deposit.

Name _____

Date _____

BANK DEPOSIT DETAIL

BANK NUMBER	PAYMENTS			
	BY CHECK OR PMO	BY COIN OR CURRENCY	CREDIT CARD	
TOTALS				

CURRENCY	
COIN	
CHECKS	
CREDIT CARDS	
TOTAL RECEIPTS	
LESS CREDIT CARD $	
TOTAL DEPOSITS	

DEPOSIT DATE: _____ FIRM: _____

Bank deposit detail.

1. Cash Receipts Total $646.68. Two dollars and 68 cents was in coins.

2. Check payments #2387 $67 and #460 $50.

3. Credit card payments: $25 and $67.

4. Insurance payment: $1374.32 (check number 309).

I. What kind of file will the manager use to keep up with monthly bills? _____

Part IV. _____

Reconcile this bank statement.

1. Your checkbook balance is $4696.96.

2. Your statement balance is $6792.79.

3. The three checks you wrote (#1837, 1838, and 1839) have not cleared. Your deposit of $2230.00 has been posted on this statement. Does the checkbook reconcile with the statement?

_____

Name _____

Date _____

Grade _____

THIS WORKSHEET IS PROVIDED TO HELP YOU BALANCE YOUR ACCOUNT

1. Go through your register and mark each check, withdrawal, Express ATM transaction, payment, deposit, or other credit listed on this statement. Be sure that your register shows any interest paid into your account, and any service charges, automatic payments, or Express Transfers withdrawn from your account during this statement period.

2. Using the chart below, list any outstanding checks, Express ATM withdrawals, payments, or any other withdrawals (including any from previous months) that are listed in your register but are not shown on this statement.

3. Balance your account by filling in the spaces below.

ITEMS OUTSTANDING		
NUMBER	**AMOUNT**	
TOTAL	**$**	

ENTER

The NEW BALANCE shown on
this statement_____ $

ADD

Any deposits listed in your register $
or transfers into your account $
which are not shown on this $
statement.   +$ _____

                              TOTAL

CALCULATE THE SUBTOTAL_____ $

SUBTRACT

The total outstanding checks and
withdrawals from the chart at left_____ -$

CALCULATE THE ENDING BALANCE

This amount should be the same
as the current balance shown in
your check register_____ $

Sample worksheet for balancing account.

CHAPTER 20

Medical Practice Management

Part I. Vocabulary

Directions: Insert the correct vocabulary term.

1. The co-workers at Diamond Family Care are a _____ group.

2. The bookkeeper who mishandled practice funds was found guilty of _____.

3. One of the _____ is a fifty-dollar bonus for perfect attendance each month.

4. Rumors abound when staff _____ is low.

5. Refusal to perform a routine duty for the office manager might be perceived as

   _____.

6. The office manager issues verbal _____ to help correct deficiencies.

Part II.

A. List six tasks performed by the medical office manager

   1. _____

   2. _____

   3. _____

   4. _____

   5. _____

   6. _____

B. Examine the notice of practice closure below. Record your thoughts about the ad and discuss with your classmates.

_____

_____

_____

_____

ince April was $6543 that the Spro anufacturing Company spent in e for Rep. Alphonse Traubin, D-NH. if Thacburn, and his wife Shakira, comlass to Vancouver, British Co-BIA for a speech at a two day con-ence. Traubin spokesman, Kevin th, also traveled to the conference an additional $1643 in travel, lodg-and meals.

Smith said that because Traubin he conference for the entire time, the expenses are legally buisness

ut they aren't allowed to pay for the ips. Atttendence at events is not mandatory. Some staffers submit tdated forms that don't indicate, as e new ones require, whether they ok their spouses or children along

hat all legal channels will be pro-ly contacted.

When the Nuclear Energy Inst-te took Galveston and the other gressional staffers to France, in see BUSINESS, B-13

Dr. Fred Davenport

announces the transfer of his practice, Diamonte Cardiology, to the Cardiology Clinic of Dobbins, Arizona.

Patients of Dr. Davenport's have had their records transferred to the offices ot the Cardiology Clinic of Dobbins, Arizona.

Dr. Davenport thanks the community and patients who have entrusted their care to him over the years. Patients are urged to continue their care at the Cardiology Clinic of Dobbins, Arizona.

Cardiology Clinic of Dobbins, Arizona (998) 775-2323

Out-of-town referrals and consultations accepted

Answering Service and 24-Hour #
(998) 775-2323

BLUE CROSS • PRIVATE INSURANCE • MEDICARE
(PARTICIPATING) • HMO and PPO PLANS ACCEPTED

Newspaper advertisement of facility closure.

C. List five essential elements of a team.

1. _____

2. _____

3. _____

4. _____

5. _____

Part III.

AGENDA FOR HIM COMMITTEE

Health Information Management Committee
Meeting: October 19, 2000

Agenda
  I. Call to order
  II. Review of minutes
  III. Old business
  IV. Record review
  V. New business
  VI. Reports
        Delinquent record count
        Quality audit of HIM functions
  VII. Adjourn

Next Meeting: November 16, 2000

Agenda for HIM committee.

Examine the agenda for the Health Information Management Committee and answer the following questions.

1. When would be an appropriate time to record attendance? _____

2. When would be an appropriate time to present a pilot staffing plan? _____

3. When would be the best time to discuss unresolved business? _____

4. What are the advantages of having a written agenda? _____

_____

_____

Part IV.

A. **Directions:** Examine the list of motivators below. Circle five motivators that are helping you to reach your educational goals.

a challenge   fulfillment

money   integrity

praise   honor

satisfaction   reputation

freedom   responsibility

fear   prestige

family   needs

insecurity   love

competition

B. **Directions:** Examine the organizational chart for a fictitious doctor's office and answer the following questions.

1. The office manager is directly supervised by whom? _____

2. The office manager has the sole responsibility for which three groups? _____

   _____

3. Why do you think that nurses and medical assistants are also supervised by the physician?

   _____

4. In this organization, do licensed practical nurses (LPNs) and licensed visiting nurses (LVNs) supervise

   medical assistants? _____

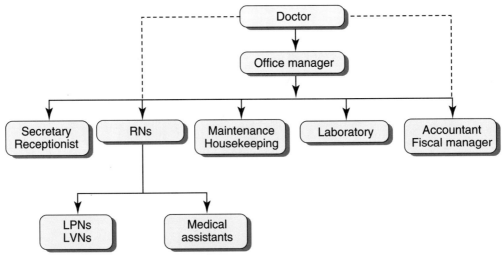

Sample of employees in a physician's office.

C. List the three types of leaders. Provide the name of a teacher, coach, or employer who fits the description of each of these types of leaders.

1. _____

2. _____

3. _____

CHAPTER 21

Medical Practice Marketing and Customer Service

Part I. Vocabulary

Directions: Insert the appropriate vocabulary word for each definition.

1. _____ Something toward which effort is directed; an aim, goal, or end of action.

2. _____ The process of using marketing and education strategies to reach and involve diverse audiences through the use of key messages and effective programs.

3. _____ The process or technique of promoting, selling, and distributing a product or service.

4. _____ The surgical or dental specialty concerned with the design, construction, and fitting of prostheses, which are artificial devices that replace missing parts of the body.

5. _____ Capable of being appraised at an actual or approximate value; capable of being precisely identified or realized by the mind.

6. _____ A specific group of individuals to whom the marketing plan is directed.

Part II.

A. List the four P's of marketing.

1. _____

2. _____

3. _____

4. _____

B. Describe the steps in developing a marketing plan.

1. _____

2. _____

3. _____

4. _____

5. _____

C. Give examples of community involvement that may promote a medical practice.

1. _____

2. _____

3. _____

D. Differentiate between advertising and public relations.

_____

_____

_____

_____

_____

E. List the eight deadly sins of customer service.

1. _____

2. _____

3. _____

4. _____

5. _____

6. _____

7. _____

8. _____

F. List the four basic steps for building a website.

1. _____

2. _____

3. _____

4. _____

Part III. _____

Directions: Visit www.aama-ntl.org and find websites for American Association of Medical Assistants affiliates in different states. Evaluate each website according to the following criteria.

Website	Overall Appeal	Content	Navigation	Font	Consistency

Part IV. _____

The patient is the most important customer in the medical practice. Name other customers in a medical practice.

1. _____

2. _____

3. _____

4. _____

CHAPTER 22

Health Information Management

Part I. Vocabulary

Directions: Match the following terms and definitions.

1. _____ Proof of; with regard to medical records, it applies to a signature, initials, or computer keystroke by the maker of the record that verifies that the record is correct.

2. _____ To manage to get around, especially by ingenuity or stratagem.

3. _____ Something, as a symptom or condition, that makes a particular treatment or procedure inadvisable.

4. _____ Containing or made up of fundamentally different and often incongruous elements; markedly distinct in quality or character.

5. _____ To convert from one system of communication to another; encode.

6. _____ Containing or characterized by error or assumption.

7. _____ Originating or taking place in a hospital.

8. _____ Activities designed to increase the quality of a product or service through process or system changes that increase efficiency or effectiveness.

9. _____ An unexpected occurrence involving death or serious physical or psychological injury, or the risk thereof.

10. _____ Established by authority, custom, or general consent as a model or example; something set up and established by authority as a rule for the measure of quantity, weight, extent, value, or quality.

11. _____ To change the relative place or normal order of; to alter the sequence.

A. disparities

B. authenticated

C. erroneous

D. transposed

E. standards

F. circumvent

G. encrypted

H. quality assurance

I. sentinel events

J. nosocomial

K. contraindications

Part II.

Phone-etics Game

Directions: Use the telephone keypad below to spell out the missing words.

A. The health information profession is supported by a national organization called the 2-4-4-6-2.

B. The 4-4-7-2-2 Act of 1996 was developed in part to help ensure the confidentiality of medical records.

C. 5-2-2-4-6 is a nonprofit organization that assists healthcare facilities by providing accreditation services.

1	ABC 2	DEF 3
GHI 4	JKL 5	MNO 6
PRS 7	TUV 8	WXY 9
*	0	#

Part III.

A medical assistant gives an injection of penicillin to a patient who reported an allergy to amoxicillin. The patient complains of itching and experiences shortness of breath and wheezing while sitting in the treatment room. The patient collapses to the floor and stops breathing. Cardiopulmonary resuscitation (CPR) is initiated, and an ambulance is called. The patient is transported on life support to the local emergency department. The patient dies 12 hours later. Complete an incident report for this sentinel event.

Incident Report
Do Not File in Medical Records

Confidential and privileged health care quality improvement information prepared in anticipation of litigation

Name: _____ Employee ☐ Patient ☐ Visitor ☐

Attending physician: _____
MR # _____ SS # _____
D.O.B. ___/___/___   Sex: M[ ] F[ ]
Admission date: ___/___/___
Primary diagnosis: _____
_____

Facility name: _____
_____
Site (if applicable) _____
City _____
Facility ID# _____
State _____
Phone # _____

SECTION I: General Information

General Identification (circle one):
001 Inpatient
002 Outpatient
003 Nonpatient
004 Equipment only

Location (circle one):
005 Bathroom/toilet
006 Beauty shop
007 Cafeteria/dining room
008 Corridor/hall
009 During transport
010 Emergency department
011 Exterior grounds
012 ICU/SCU/CCU
013 Labor/delivery/birthing
014 Nursery
015 Outpatient clinic
016 Patient room
017 Radiology
018 Recovery room
019 Recreation area
020 Rehab
021 Shower room
022 Surgical suite
023 Treatment/exam room

Treatment Rendered (circle one):
024 Emergency room
025 First aid
026 None
026 Transfer to other facility
027 X-ray

SECTION II: Nature of Incident   (Circle all that apply):

001 Adverse outcome after surgery or anesthetic
002 Anaphylactic shock
003 Anoxic event
004 Apgar score of 5 or less
005 Aspiration
006 Assault or altercation/combative event
007 Blood or IV variance
008 Blood/body fluid exposure
009 Code/arrest
010 Damage/loss of organ
011 Death
012 Dental-related complication
013 Dissatisfaction/noncompliance*
014 Equipment operation*
015 Fall with injury*
016 Fall without injury*
017 Handling of and/or exposure to hazardous waste
018 Informed consent issue
019 Injury to other
020 Injury to self
021 Loss of limb
022 Loss of vision
023 Medication variance*
024 Needle puncture/sharp injury
025 Paralysis
026 Patient-to-patient altercation
027 Perinatal complication*
028 Poisoning
029 Suspected nonstaff-to-patient abuse
030 Suspected staff-to-patient abuse
031 Thermal burn
032 Treatment/procedure issue
033 Ulcer: nosocomial stage III/IV

* Complete appropriate area in Section III

SECTION III: Type of Incident

If death, circle all that apply:
001 After medical equipment failure
002 After power equipment failure or damage
003 During surgery or postanesthesia
004 Within 24 hours of admission to facility
005 Within 1 week of fall in facility
006 Within 24 hours of medication error

Blood/IV Variance Issues (circle all that apply):
007 Additive
008 Administration consent
009 Contraindications/allergies
010 Equipment malfunction
011 Infusion rate
012 Labeling issue
013 Reaction
014 Solution/blood type
015 Transcription
016 Patient identification
017 Allergic/adverse reaction
018 Infiltration
019 Phlebitis

Dissatisfaction/Noncompliance (circle all that apply):
020 AMA
021 Elopement
022 Irate or angry (either family or patient)
023 Left without service
024 Noncompliant patient
025 Refused prescribed treatment

Falls (circle all that apply):*
001 Assisted fall
002 Found on floor
003 From bed
004 From chair
005 From commode/toilet
006 From exam table
007 From stretcher
008 From wheelchair
009 Patient states—unwitnessed
010 Unassisted fall
011 While ambulating
012 Witnessed fall

* For any marks in this field, Section V must be completed

Medication Variance Issues (circle all that apply):
013 Contraindication/allergies
014 Delay in dispensing
015 Incorrect dose
016 Expired drug
017 Medication identification
018 Narcotic log variance
019 Not ordered
020 Ordered, not given
021 Patient identification
022 Reaction
023 Route
024 Rx incorrectly dispensed
025 Time of dose
026 Transcription

Incident report.

Part IV.

Evaluate the confidentiality statement for Diamonte Hospital. Reword the statement to make it appropriate for a medical practice setting. Indicate your proposed changes on the confidentiality statement.

DIAMONTE
HOSPITAL

Diamonte, Arizona 89104 • TEL. 602-484-9991

CONFIDENTIALITY STATEMENT

I, _____ , understand that in the course of my activities/business at or for Diamonte Hospital, I am required to have access to and am involved in the viewing, reviewing, and/or processing of patient care data and/or health information.

I understand that I am obligated by State Law, Federal Law, and Diamonte Hospital to maintain the confidentiality of these data and information at all times.

I understand that a violation of these confidentiality considerations may result in punitive legal action against me.

I certify by my signature below that this Confidentiality Statement has been explained to me, and I agree to the principles contained herein as a condition of my activity/business at or for Diamonte Hospital.

_____
Signature/date

_____
Witness/date

Confidentiality statement.

CHAPTER 23

Management of Practice Finances

Part I. Vocabulary

Directions: Define the following.

1. Assets

_____

_____

2. Accounts payable

_____

_____

3. Accounts receivable

_____

_____

4. Accounts receivable trial balance

_____

_____

5. Accrual basis of accounting

_____

_____

6. Balance sheet

_____

_____

7. Bookkeeping

_____

_____

8. Cash basis of accounting

_____

_____

9. Cash flow statement

_____

_____

10. Disbursements journal

_____

_____

11. Equities

_____

_____

12. Fiscal year

_____

_____

13. In balance

_____

_____

14. Invoice

_____

_____

15. Liabilities

_____

_____

16. Packing slip

_____

_____

17. Petty cash fund

_____

_____

18. Statement

_____

_____

19. Statement of income and expense

_____

_____

20. Trial balance

_____

_____

Part II. _____

A. Differentiate between accounting and bookkeeping.

_____

_____

_____

B. List three cardinal rules of bookkeeping.

1. _____

2. _____

3. _____

C. Name three types of bookkeeping systems commonly used in medical offices.

1. _____

2. _____

3. _____

D. List three drawbacks to a single-entry system.

1. _____

2. _____

3. _____

Part III. _____

A. Give examples of accounts that are commonly set up for practice disbursements in a pegboard system.

1. _____

2. _____

3. _____

4. _____

5. _____

6. _____

7. _____

8. _____

9. _____

10. _____

11. _____

B. Complete two purchase orders using an office supply catalog, newspaper ad, or the Internet. Complete one purchase order for supplies (things that are used up on a routine basis); complete the other for equipment (things that are re-usable and usually of value).

Name _____

Date _____

PURCHASE ORDER   No. 1554

Bill to: **Ship to:**

Blackburn Primary Care Associates. PC   Blackburn Primary Care Associates, PC
1990 Turquoise Drive   1990 Turquoise Drive
Blackburn, WI 54937   Blackburn, WI 54937

Vendor: _____

Terms: _____

ORDER #	DESCRIPTION	QTY.	COLOR	SIZE	UNIT PRICE	TOTAL PRICE
					SUBTOTAL	
					TAX	
					SHIPPING	
					TOTAL	

Purchase order.

Name _____

Date _____

PURCHASE ORDER   No. _1554_

Bill to: **Ship to:**

Blackburn Primary Care Associates. PC   Blackburn Primary Care Associates, PC
1990 Turquoise Drive   1990 Turquoise Drive
Blackburn, WI 54937   Blackburn, WI 54937

Vendor: _____

_____

_____

Terms: _____

ORDER #	DESCRIPTION	QTY.	COLOR	SIZE	UNIT PRICE	TOTAL PRICE
					SUBTOTAL	
					TAX	
					SHIPPING	
					TOTAL	

Part IV.

A. Your manager asks you to go by the local discount store and purchase sponges for the housekeeper. Your receipt totals $4.37. Complete this petty cash request form for reimbursement.

Petty Cash Request

$25 Limit

Receipt must be attached

Date: _____

For: _____

Approved by: _____

Amount: _____ Receipt attached _____

Signature of person receiving reimbursement:

_____

B. The manager notices that there is less than $10 in the petty cash box. How will the manager replace these funds?

_____

_____

_____

_____

C. Complete the checks below. The beginning balance is $3245.62.

1. Fifty dollars for the petty cash box.

2. Malpractice Insurance Company of America: $1250.00.

3. Pay the Forms-R-Us bill for $147.82, but first show a deposit for $882.17.

4. What is the final balance?

Name _____

Date _____

1837

DATE _____
TO _____
FOR _____

BALANCE BROUGHT FORWARD		
DEPOSITS		
BALANCE		
AMT THIS CK		
BALANCE CARRIED FORWARD		

BLACKBURN PRIMARY CARE ASSOCIATES, PC
1990 Turquoise Drive
Blackburn, WI 54937
608-459-8857

1837
94-72/1224

DATE _____

PAY TO THE ORDER OF _____ $ _____

_____ DOLLARS

DERBYSHIRE SAVINGS
Member FDIC
P.O. BOX 8923
Blackburn, WI 54937

FOR _____

⑈055003⑈ 446782011⑈ 678800470

1838

DATE _____
TO _____
FOR _____

BALANCE BROUGHT FORWARD		
DEPOSITS		
BALANCE		
AMT THIS CK		
BALANCE CARRIED FORWARD		

BLACKBURN PRIMARY CARE ASSOCIATES, PC
1990 Turquoise Drive
Blackburn, WI 54937
608-459-8857

1838
94-72/1224

DATE _____

PAY TO THE ORDER OF _____ $ _____

_____ DOLLARS

DERBYSHIRE SAVINGS
Member FDIC
P.O. BOX 8923
Blackburn, WI 54937

FOR _____

⑈055003⑈ 446782011⑈ 678800470

1839

DATE _____
TO _____
FOR _____

BALANCE BROUGHT FORWARD		
DEPOSITS		
BALANCE		
AMT THIS CK		
BALANCE CARRIED FORWARD		

BLACKBURN PRIMARY CARE ASSOCIATES, PC
1990 Turquoise Drive
Blackburn, WI 54937
608-459-8857

1839
94-72/1224

DATE _____

PAY TO THE ORDER OF _____ $ _____

_____ DOLLARS

DERBYSHIRE SAVINGS
Member FDIC
P.O. BOX 8923
Blackburn, WI 54937

FOR _____

⑈055003⑈ 446782011⑈ 678800470

D. Describe the following.

1. SS-5 _____

2. W-2 _____

3. W-3 _____

4. W-4 _____

CHAPTER **24**

Assisting with Medical Emergencies

Part I. Vocabulary

A. **Directions:** Define the following.

1. cyanosis _____

2. dyspnea _____

3. ecchymosis _____

4. emetic _____

5. fibrillation _____

6. hematuria _____

7. mediastinum _____

8. myocardium _____

9. necrosis _____

10. photophobia _____

11. polydipsia _____

12. polyuria _____

13. transient ischemic attack _____

B. **Directions:** Fill in the blanks with the correct terms.

1. _____ _____ is defined as the immediate care given to a person who has been injured or has suddenly taken ill.

2. AED stands for _____.

3. CPR stands for _____.

4. CVA stands for _____.

5. TIA stands for _____.

6. MI stands for _____.

7. A heart attack, or _____, is usually caused by a blockage of the coronary arteries, which decreases the amount of blood being delivered to the myocardium. The most common signal of a heart attack is an uncomfortable pressure, squeezing, fullness, or pain in the center of the chest.

C. List five other symptoms of a heart attack.

1. _____

2. _____

3. _____

4. _____

5. _____

D. List seven types of shock.

1. _____

2. _____

3. _____

4. _____

5. _____

6. _____

7. _____

E. Sprains and strains are treated with:

1. _____

2. _____

3. _____

F. Give five examples of situations in which patients with abdominal pain should be seen immediately.

1. _____

2. _____

3. _____

4. _____

5. _____

Part II. Heat-Related Illnesses

Directions: Fill in the blanks with the correct terms.

1. _____ _____ is the most dangerous form of heat-related injury and results in a shutdown of body systems.

2. _____ are the initial signs of a heat-related emergency, and heat exhaustion is a more serious condition.

3. Patients with _____ _____ appear flushed and report headaches, nausea, vertigo, and weakness.

Part III. Emergency Situations

Directions: Complete the table with appropriate triage questions and home care advice.

Situation	Triage Questions	Home Care Advice
Syncope	1. 2.	1. 2. 3.
Animal bites	1. 2. 3.	1. 2. 3.
Insect bites and stings	1. 2.	1. 2. 3.
Asthma	1. 2.	1.
Burns	1. 2. 3.	1. 2. 3. 4.

Situation	Triage Questions	Home Care Advice
Wounds	1. 2. 3. 4.	1. 2. 3. 4.
Head injury	1.	1.

Chapter 24 Quiz

Name: _____

1. AED stands for _____

   _____ _____.

2. A _____ _____
   seizure involves uncontrolled muscular
   contractions.

3. List three symptoms of a heart attack.

   a. _____

   b. _____

   c. _____

4. Syncope means to _____.

5. List three causes of shock.

   a. _____

   b. _____

   c. _____

6. True or False: Epinephrine is a
   vasoconstrictor.

7. True or False: Accidental poisoning is the
   leading cause of death in children.

8. List two ways to treat lacerations.

   a. _____

   b. _____

9. During a life-threatening emergency,

   always call _____.

10. _____ means to sort patients.

CHAPTER **25**

Career Development and Life Skills

Part I. Vocabulary

Directions: Match the following terms and definitions.

1. _____ To give an expert judgment of the value or merit of; in this chapter, the evaluation of work performance.

2. _____ A return offer made by one who has rejected an offer or job.

3. _____ A failure to pay financial debts, especially a student loan.

4. _____ A postponement, especially of repayment of a student loan.

5. _____ Expressing sincerity and honest feeling.

6. _____ Not tolerable or bearable.

7. _____ To imitate or practice.

8. _____ The exchange of information or services among individuals, groups, or institutions; in this chapter, it involves meeting and getting to know individuals in the same or similar career fields and sharing information about available opportunities.

9. _____ Having a clear decisive relevance to the matter in hand.

10. _____ To read and mark corrections.

11. _____ Something produced by a cause or necessarily following from a set of conditions.

12. _____ To correct by removing errors.

13. _____ Having or marked by keen insight and ability to penetrate deeply and thoroughly.

14. _____ Marked by compact, precise expression without wasted words.

15. _____ A condensed statement or outline.

16. _____ The work in which a person is regularly employed.

A. succinct

B. counteroffer

C. synopsis

D. appraisals

E. rectify

F. proofread

G. intolerable

H. default

I. pertinent

J. ramification

K. networking

L. vocation

M. subtle

N. genuineness

O. mock

P. deferment

Part II.

A. **Directions:** List nine methods of job searching.

1. _____

2. _____

3. _____

4. _____

5. _____

6. _____

7. _____

8. _____

9. _____

B. **Directions:** Complete the job application that is included in this workbook. Use factual information. Remember: Neatness counts.

C. **Directions:** Prepare a draft resume using the blank pages included in this chapter.

DIAMONTE
HOSPITAL

APPLICATION FOR EMPLOYMENT

This application is not a contract. It is intended to provide information for evaluating your suitability for employment. Please read each question carefully and give an honest and complete answer. Qualified applicants receive consideration for employment without unlawful discrimination because of sex, religion, race, color, national origin, age, disability, or other classification protected by law. Applications will remain active for three months.

PLEASE TYPE OR PRINT ALL INFORMATION

Date: _____

Position(s) applying for: _____

How did you learn about us? ☐ Walk-in ☐ Friend ☐ Relative ☐ Job hotline ☐ Employee ☐ Other
☐ Advertisement (Please state name of publication) _____ Referred by: _____

Name: _____
              Last   *First*   *Middle initial*

Mailing address: _____
                 City   *State*   *Zip code*

Phone: (_____) _____   (_____) _____   Social Security #: _____
      Home   *Message*

If related to anyone in our employ, state name and department: _____

If you have been employed under another name, please list here: _____

Are you under 18 years of age? .... ☐ Yes   ☐ No

Are you currently employed? .... ☐ Yes   ☐ No

May we contact your present employer? .... ☐ Yes   ☐ No

Do you have legal rights to work in this country?
  (Proof of legal rights to work in this country will be required upon employment) ... ☐ Yes   ☐ No

Have you ever been employed with us before? .... ☐ Yes   ☐ No *If "yes," give date(s):* _____

Are you available to work: .... ☐ Full-time ☐ Part-time ☐ Shift work ☐ Temporary

Are you available to work overtime if required? .... ☐ Yes   ☐ No

How flexible are you in accepting varying scheduled hours? .... ☐ Very flexible ☐ Somewhat flexible
                                            ☐ Need set schedule

Minimum salary desired: _____

Have you ever been discharged from a job or forced to resign? .... ☐ Yes   ☐ No
  Explain: _____

Have you ever been convicted of a felony?
  If "yes," please explain: .... ☐ Yes ☐ No
  Criminal convictions are not an absolute bar to _____
  employment but will be considered with respect
  to the specific requirements of the job for which _____
  you are applying. _____

EDUCATION

High school: _____ High school graduate/GED: ☐Yes ☐No
_____ Date:_____

College:_____ Graduated: ☐Yes ☐No

Major/field(s) of study: _____ Degree: _____
Date:_____

College: _____ Graduated: ☐Yes ☐No

Major/field(s) of study: _____ Degree: _____
Date:_____

Technical, business, or
correspondence school: _____ Graduated: ☐Yes ☐No

Major/field(s) of study: _____ Degree: _____
Date:_____

Describe any specialized training, apprenticeship, and skills such as computer, office equipment, etc. _____
_____
_____
_____
_____

LICENSES AND CERTIFICATIONS

Type of license(s)/certification(s): _____ Expiration date: _____
Type of license(s)/certification(s): _____ Expiration date: _____
Type of license(s)/certification(s): _____ Expiration date: _____
Verified by: _____
Date:_____

REFERENCES

(Give name, address, and telephone number of three references that you have known for at least one year who are not related to you.)

Name: _____ Phone:_____ Years acquainted:_____
Address: _____ Business: _____

Name: _____ Phone:_____ Years acquainted:_____
Address: _____ Business: _____

Name: _____ Phone:_____ Years acquainted:_____
Address: _____ Business: _____

EMPLOYMENT EXPERIENCE

(Please list all employment experience, with most recent employment first. If more space is needed, please use the Additional Employment form.)

Employer: _____ Duties and skills performed: _____
Address: _____ _____
Phone number(s) _____ _____
Job title: _____ _____
Supervisor's name/title: _____ _____
Reason for leaving: _____ _____
Salary received: _____ hourly / weekly / monthly _____
Employed from: _____ to _____
       month / year   *month / year*

Employer: _____ Duties and skills performed: _____
Address: _____ _____
Phone number(s) _____ _____
Job title: _____ _____
Supervisor's name/title: _____ _____
Reason for leaving: _____ _____
Salary received: _____ hourly / weekly / monthly _____
Employed from: _____ to _____
       month / year   *month / year*

Employer: _____ Duties and skills performed: _____
Address: _____ _____
Phone number(s) _____ _____
Job title: _____ _____
Supervisor's name/title: _____ _____
Reason for leaving: _____ _____
Salary received: _____ hourly / weekly / monthly _____
Employed from: _____ to _____
       month / year   *month / year*

Do you expect any of the employers listed above to give you a poor reference? ☐ Yes ☐ No
If yes, explain: _____
_____

APPLICANT'S STATEMENT

I hereby certify that the statements and information provided are true, and I understand that any false statements or omissions are cause for termination. I agree to submit to a drug test and physical following any conditional offer of employment, and I grant permission to Diamonte Hospital to investigate my criminal history, education, prior employment history, and references, and hereby release all persons or agencies from all liability or any damage for issuing this information.

I understand that this application is current for only **three months**. At the end of that time, if I do not hear from Diamonte Hospital and still wish to be considered for employment, it will be necessary to update my application.

_____   _____
Signature of Applicant   *Date*

_____
Print Name

DIAMONTE
HOSPITAL

Draft Resumé

Draft Resumé

Part III.

Directions: Evaluate Teresa O'Sullivan's cover letter. Describe what you like about the letter and make notes of additional information that you would include in your own cover letter.

Theresa O'Sullivan
233 Wentworth Street, San Diego, CA 92100
Telephone (619) 222-3333

June 15, 20xx

Arthur M. Blackburn, MD
2200 Broadway
Any Town, US 98765

Dear Doctor Blackburn:

In a few weeks, I will complete my formal training in medical assisting with an Associate in Science degree from Ola Vista Community College.

The medical assisting program at Ola Vista includes theory and practical application in both administrative and clinical skills. My six-week supervised externship gave me additional practical experience in two specialty practices.

While studying at Ola Vista, I also worked part-time for a physician in family practice, while maintaining a 3.5 grade point average. My experience as Dr. Madden's employee is outlined on the enclosed resumé. I have enjoyed my work in Dr. Madden's office and am now seeking full-time employment.

If you will require a replacement or addition to your staff in the near future, may I be considered as an applicant? I will follow up with a telephone call within a week.

Sincerely yours,

Theresa O'Sullivan

Enc. Resumé

Part IV.

A. **Directions:** Set some realistic goals for your career in medical assisting by answering the following questions.

1. Where am I today?

_____

_____

_____

_____

_____

_____

2. Where will I be in five years?

_____

_____

_____

_____

_____

_____

3. Where will I be in ten years?

_____

_____

_____

_____

_____

_____

4. What additional skills do I need to get where I want to be?

_____

_____

_____

_____

_____

_____

B. **Directions:** Plan a budget for yourself using your actual living expenses.

The Guideline Budget

MONTHLY INCOME	AMOUNT
Net Income	
Spouse Net Income	
Child Support	
Other Income	

MONTHLY EXPENSES	AMOUNT
Rent	
Gas	
Electric	
Home/Renters Insurance	
Water/Sewage	
Trash	
Home Telephone	
Cell Telephone	
Pager	
Cable TV/Satellite	
Internet/DSL	
Child Care	
Lawn Care	
Clothing	
Food-Home	
Food-Work or School	
Food-Eating Out	
Laundry/Dry Cleaning	
Medical Expenses	
Dental Expenses	
Life Insurance	
Medical Insurance	
Dental Insurance	
Eyeglasses	
Prescriptions	
Automobile Payment	
Automobile Insurance	
Repairs	
Gas/Oil	
Furniture	
Beauty/Barber Shop	
Pet Expenses	
Student Loan	
Others Loans	
Credit Cards	
Church/charities	
Birthdays	
Anniversaries	
Christmas	
Vacation Planning	
Entertainment	

Procedure Checklists

Student Name _____ Date _____ Score _____

Procedure 9-1 Answering the Telephone

Task: To answer the phone in a professional manner, respond to a request for action, and accurately record a message.

Equipment and Supplies:
- Telephone
- Message pad
- Pen or pencil
- Appointment book
- Script for conversation

Standards: Complete the procedure and all critical steps in _____ minutes with a minimum

score of _____ % within three attempts.

Scoring: Divide points earned by total possible points. Failure to perform a critical step that is indicated with an asterisk (*), will result in an unsatisfactory overall score.

Time began _____ **Time ended** _____

Steps	Possible Points	First Attempt	Second Attempt	Third Attempt
1. Answer the phone after the first ring and before the third ring, speaking directly into the transmitter, with the mouthpiece 1 inch from the mouth.	20			
2. Speak distinctly with a pleasant tone and expression, at a moderate rate, and with sufficient volume. Remember to smile.	10			
3. Identify yourself and the office.*	20			
4. Verify the identity of the caller.	10			
5. Provide the caller with the requested information or service, if possible.	10			
6. Take a message for further action, if required.	20			
7. Terminate the call in a pleasant manner and replace the receiver gently.	10			

Documentation in the Medical Record

_____

_____

_____

_____

Comments:

Total Points Earned _____ Divided by _____ Total Possible Points = _____ % Score

Instructor's Signature _____

Student Name _____ Date _____ Score _____

Procedure 9-2 Taking a Message

Task: To take an accurate telephone message and follow up on the requests made by the caller.

Equipment and Supplies:
- Telephone
- Message pad
- Pen or pencil
- Notepad

Standards: Complete the procedure and all critical steps in _____ minutes with a minimum

score of _____ % within three attempts.

Scoring: Divide points earned by total possible points. Failure to perform a critical step that is indicated with an asterisk (*), will result in an unsatisfactory overall score.

Time began _____ **Time ended** _____

Steps	Possible Points	First Attempt	Second Attempt	Third Attempt
1. Answer the telephone using the guidelines in Procedure 9-1, Answering the Telephone.	10	_____	_____	_____
2. Using a message pad or notepad, take the phone message, obtaining the following information: a. the name of the person to whom the call is directed b. the name of the person calling c. the caller's daytime and/or telephone number d. the reason for the call e. the action to be taken f. the date and time of the call g. the initials of the person taking the call	20	_____	_____	_____
3. Repeat the information back to the caller after the message is recorded on the message pad.	10	_____	_____	_____
4. Provide the caller with an approximation of the time and date that he or she will be called back, if possible.	10	_____	_____	_____
5. End the call and wait for the caller to hang up first.	10	_____	_____	_____
6. Deliver the phone message to the appropriate person. Separate trays or slots for each staff member are helpful.	10	_____	_____	_____
7. Follow up on important messages.	10	_____	_____	_____

Steps	Possible Points	First Attempt	Second Attempt	Third Attempt
8. Keep old message books for future reference. Carbonless copies will allow the facility to keep a permanent record of phone messages.	10			
9. File pertinent phone messages in the patient's chart.	10			

Comments:

Total Points Earned _____ Divided by _____ Total Possible Points = _____ % Score

Instructor's Signature _____

Student Name _____ Date _____ Score _____

Procedure 9-3 Calling Pharmacy with New or Refill Prescription Orders

Task: To call in an accurate prescription to the pharmacy for a patient in the most efficient manner.

Equipment and Supplies:
- Prescription
- Notepad
- Patient chart
- Telephone

Standards: Complete the procedure and all critical steps in _____ minutes with a minimum

score of _____ % within three attempts.

Scoring: Divide points earned by total possible points. Failure to perform a critical step that is indicated with an asterisk (*), will result in an unsatisfactory overall score.

Time began _____ **Time ended** _____

Steps	Possible Points	First Attempt	Second Attempt	Third Attempt
1. Receive the call from the patient requesting a prescription, using appropriate telephone technique.	10			
2. Obtain the following information from the patient: a. patient's name b. telephone number where he or she can be reached c. patient's symptoms and current condition d. history of this condition e. treatments the patient has tried f. pharmacy name and telephone number	20			
3. Write the prescription in the patient's chart that the physician wishes the patient to have. Be very careful to transcribe the information correctly. Read it back to the physician.	10			
4. If the prescription is a refill, give the physician the patient's chart with the message requesting a refill attached, along with the information in procedure step two as listed above.	10			
5. Note the comments that the physician writes in the chart. If the prescription is written or a refill is approved, call the patient's pharmacy and ask to speak to a member of the pharmacy staff.	10			
6. Ask the pharmacy staff member to repeat the prescription back to you.	10			

Steps	Possible Points	First Attempt	Second Attempt	Third Attempt
7. Note the date and time that the prescription was called to the pharmacy in the chart.	10			
8. Call the patient to notify him or her that the prescription has been called in. Provide any information regarding the prescription doses, frequency, etc. that is requested by the physician. Tell the patient when to return to the office, if necessary. Ask the patient to write this information down.	20			

Comments:

Total Points Earned _____ Divided by _____ Total Possible Points = _____ % Score

Instructor's Signature _____

Procedure 10-1 Preparing and Maintaining the Appointment Book

Task: To establish the matrix of the appointment page, arrange appointments for one day, and enter information.

Equipment and Supplies:
- Page from appointment book
- Office policy for office hours and doctors' availability
- Clerical supplies
- Calendar
- Description of patients to be scheduled

Standards: Complete the procedure and all critical steps in _____ minutes with a minimum

score of _____ % within three attempts.

Scoring: Divide points earned by total possible points. Failure to perform a critical step that is indicated with an asterisk (*), will result in an unsatisfactory overall score.

Time began _____ **Time ended** _____

Steps	Possible Points	First Attempt	Second Attempt	Third Attempt
1. Identify each patient's complaint.	15			
2. Establish the matrix of the appointment page for the day.	15			
3. Consult guidelines to determine the length of time necessary for each patient.	15			
4. Allot appointment time according to the complaint and facilities available.*	25			
5. Enter information in the appointment book. NOTE: A telephone number must follow the patient's name. If the patient is new, add the letters NP (new patient) after his or her name.	15			
6. Allow buffer time in the morning and afternoon.	15			

Comments:

Total Points Earned _____ Divided by _____ Total Possible Points = _____ % Score

Instructor's Signature _____

Procedure 10-2 Scheduling a New Patient

Task: To schedule a new patient for a first office visit.

Equipment and Supplies:
- Appointment book
- Scheduling guidelines
- Appointment card
- Telephone

Standards: Complete the procedure and all critical steps in _____ minutes with a minimum

score of _____ % within three attempts.

Scoring: Divide points earned by total possible points. Failure to perform a critical step that is indicated with an asterisk (*), will result in an unsatisfactory overall score.

Time began _____ **Time ended** _____

Steps	Possible Points	First Attempt	Second Attempt	Third Attempt
1. Obtain the patient's full name, birth date, address, and telephone number. NOTE: Verify the spelling of the name.	10			
2. Determine whether the patient was referred by another physician.	10			
3. Determine the patient's chief complaint and when the first symptoms occurred.*	20			
4. Search the appointment book for the first suitable appointment time and an alternate time.	10			
5. Offer the patient a choice of these dates and times.	10			
6. Enter the mutually agreed-upon time in the appointment book, followed by the patient's telephone number. NOTE: Indicate that the patient is new by adding the letters NP.	15			
7. If new patients are expected to pay at the time of the visit, explain this financial arrangement when the appointment is made.	10			
8. Offer travel directions for reaching the office and parking instructions.	5			
9. Repeat the day, and time of the appointment before saying good-bye to the patient.	10			

Comments:

Total Points Earned _____ Divided by _____ Total Possible Points = _____ % Score

Instructor's Signature _____

Student Name _____ Date _____ Score _____

Procedure 10-3 Scheduling Outpatient Admissions and Procedures

Task: To schedule a patient for an outpatient diagnostic test ordered by a physician within the time frame needed by the physician, confirm the appointment with the patient, and issue all required instructions.

Equipment and Supplies:
- Diagnostic test order from physician
- Name, address, and telephone number of diagnostic facility
- Patient chart
- Test preparation instructions
- Telephone

Standards: Complete the procedure and all critical steps in _____ minutes with a minimum

score of _____ % within three attempts.

Scoring: Divide points earned by total possible points. Failure to perform a critical step that is indicated with an asterisk (*), will result in an unsatisfactory overall score.

Time began _____ Time ended _____

Steps	Possible Points	First Attempt	Second Attempt	Third Attempt
1. Obtain an oral or written order from the physician for the exact procedure to be performed.	10			
2. Determine the patient's availability.	10			
3. Telephone the diagnostic facility. • Order the specific test needed. • Establish the date and time. • Give the name, age, address, and telephone number of the patient. • Determine any special instructions for the patient. • Notify the facility of any urgency for test results.	25			
4. Notify the patient of the arrangements, including: • Name, address, and telephone number of the diagnostic facility. • Date and time to report for the test. • Instructions concerning preparation for the test (e.g., eating restrictions, fluids, medications, enemas). • Ask the patient to repeat the instructions.	25			
5. Note arrangements on the patient's chart below.	20			
6. Place reminder in a "tickler" file or on a desk calendar.	10			

Documentation in the Medical Record

_____

_____

_____

_____

Comments:

Total Points Earned _____ Divided by _____ Total Possible Points = _____ % Score

Instructor's Signature _____

Procedure 10-4 Scheduling Inpatient Admissions

Task: To schedule a patient for inpatient admission within the time frame needed by physician, confirm with the patient, and issue all required instructions.

Equipment and Supplies:
- Admissions orders from physician
- Name, address, and telephone number of inpatient facility
- Patient demographic information
- Patient chart
- Any preparation instructions for the patient
- Telephone
- Admission packet for the patient

Standards: Complete the procedure and all critical steps in _____ minutes with a minimum

score of _____ % within three attempts.

Scoring: Divide points earned by total possible points. Failure to perform a critical step that is indicated with an asterisk (*), will result in an unsatisfactory overall score.

Time began _____ **Time ended** _____

Steps	Possible Points	First Attempt	Second Attempt	Third Attempt
1. Obtain an oral or written order from the physician for the admission.	10			
2. Precertify the admission with the patient's insurance company, if necessary.	20			
3. Determine the physician and patient availability if the admission is not an emergency.	10			
4. Telephone the diagnostic facility and schedule the admission. • Order any specific tests needed. • Provide the patient's admitting diagnosis. • Establish the date and time. • Convey the patient's room preferences. • Give the name, age, address, and telephone number of the patient. • Provide the demographic information for the patient, including insurance policy numbers and addresses for filing claims. • Determine any special instructions for the patient. • Notify the facility of any urgency for test results.	20			

Steps	Possible Points	First Attempt	Second Attempt	Third Attempt
5. Notify the patient of the arrangements, including: • Name, address, and telephone number of the facility. • Date and time to report for admission. • Instructions concerning preparation for any procedures, if necessary (e.g., eating restrictions, fluids, medications, enemas) • Tell what preadmission testing will be necessary, if any. • Ask the patient to repeat the instructions.	20	_____	_____	_____
6. Note arrangements and the admission on the patient's chart.	10	_____	_____	_____
7. Place reminder on the physician's tickler or desk calendar, if needed. Be sure the information is listed on the office schedule. If the physician keeps a list of all inpatients, add the patient's name to that list.	10	_____	_____	_____

Comments:

Total Points Earned _____ Divided by _____ Total Possible Points = _____ % Score

Instructor's Signature _____

Procedure 10-5 Scheduling Inpatient Surgical Procedures

Task: To schedule a patient for inpatient surgery within the time frame needed by physician, confirm with the patient, and issue all required instructions.

Equipment and Supplies:
- Orders from physician
- Name, address, and telephone number of inpatient facility
- Patient demographic information
- Patient chart
- Any preparation instructions for the patient
- Telephone

Standards: Complete the procedure and all critical steps in _____ minutes with a minimum score of _____ % within three attempts.

Scoring: Divide points earned by total possible points. Failure to perform a critical step that is indicated with an asterisk (*), will result in an unsatisfactory overall score.

Time began _____ **Time ended** _____

Steps	Possible Points	First Attempt	Second Attempt	Third Attempt
1. Obtain an oral or written order from the physician for the admission.	10			
2. Precertify the admission with the patient's insurance company, if necessary.	10			
3. Determine the physician availability if the surgery is not an emergency. Another physician may be the surgeon. If this is the case, the surgery will need to be coordinated with his or her office as well.	10			
4. Telephone the hospital surgical department and schedule the procedure. • Order any specific tests needed. • Provide the patient's admitting diagnosis. • Establish the date and time. • Give the name, age, address, and telephone number of the patient. • Provide the demographic information for the patient, including insurance policy numbers and addresses for filing claims. • Determine any special instructions for the patient. • Notify the facility of any urgency for the surgery.	20			

Steps	Possible Points	First Attempt	Second Attempt	Third Attempt
5. Notify the patient of the arrangements, if the patient is not already admitted to the hospital. Include: • Name, address, and telephone number of the facility. • Date and time to report for admission. • Instructions concerning preparation for any procedures, if necessary (e.g., eating restrictions, fluids, medications, enemas) • Tell what preadmission testing will be necessary, if any. • Ask the patient to repeat the instructions.	20	_____	_____	_____
6. The physician should review the consent form with the patient. Have the patient sign a consent for the surgical procedure. Keep the original consent in the patient's chart and give a copy to the patient.	10	_____	_____	_____
7. Note arrangements on the patient's chart.	10	_____	_____	_____
8. Place reminder on the physician's tickler or desk calendar, if needed. Be sure the information is listed on the office schedule. If the physician keeps a list of all inpatients, add the patient's name to that list. Follow up with the hospital after the procedure regarding the patient's condition as required by the physician.	10	_____	_____	_____

Comments:

Total Points Earned _____ Divided by _____ Total Possible Points = _____ % Score

Instructor's Signature _____

Procedure 11-1 Preparing Charts for Scheduled Patients

Task: To prepare patient charts for the daily appointment schedule and have them ready for the physician before the patients' arrival.

Equipment and Supplies:
- Appointment schedule for current date
- Patient files
- Clerical supplies (e.g., pen, tape, stapler)

Standards: Complete the procedure and all critical steps in _____ minutes with a minimum

score of _____ % within three attempts.

Scoring: Divide points earned by total possible points. Failure to perform a critical step that is indicated with an asterisk (*), will result in an unsatisfactory overall score.

Time began _____ **Time ended** _____

Steps	Possible Points	First Attempt	Second Attempt	Third Attempt
1. Review the appointment schedule.	10			
2. Identify full name of each scheduled patient.	10			
3. Pull patients' charts for files, checking each patient's name on your list as each is pulled.*	10			
4. Review each chart to insure that: • All information has been correctly entered. • Any previously ordered tests have been performed and the results mounted permanently in the chart. • The results have been entered on the chart. • Replenish forms inside the chart, such as progress notes, etc.	40			
5. Annotate the appointment list with any special concerns.	10			
6. Arrange the charts sequentially according to each patient's appointment.	10			
7. Place the charts in the appropriate examination room or other specified location.	10			

Comments:

Total Points Earned _____ Divided by _____ Total Possible Points = _____ % Score

Instructor's Signature _____

Procedure 11-2 Registering a New Patient

Task: To complete a registration form for a new patient with information for credit and insurance claims, and to inform and orient the patient to the facility.

Equipment and Supplies:
• Registration form
• Clerical supplies (pen, clipboard)
• Private conference area

Standards: Complete the procedure and all critical steps in _____ minutes with a minimum

score of _____ % within three attempts.

Scoring: Divide points earned by total possible points. Failure to perform a critical step that is indicated with an asterisk (*), will result in an unsatisfactory overall score.

Time began _____ **Time ended** _____

Steps	Possible Points	First Attempt	Second Attempt	Third Attempt
1. Determine whether the patient is new.	10			
2. Obtain and record the necessary information: • Full name, birth date, name of spouse (if married) • Home address, telephone number (include ZIP and area codes) • Occupation, name of employer, business address, telephone number • Social Security number and driver's license number, if any • Name of referring physician, if any • Name and address of person responsible for payment • Method of payment • Health insurance information (photocopy both sides of insurance ID card) • Name of primary carrier • Type of coverage • Group policy number • Subscriber number • Assignment of benefits, if required	50			
3. Review the enter form and confirm patient eligibility for insurance coverage.	10			
4. Determine that required referrals have been received, if applicable.	10			
5. Explain medical and financial procedures to patients.*	10			
6. Collect copays or balance payment charges.	10			

Comments:

Total Points Earned _____ Divided by _____ Total Possible Points = _____ % Score

Instructor's Signature _____

Procedure 12-1 Composing Business Correspondence

Task: To compose a letter that will convey information in an accurate and concise manner, which is easy to comprehend by the reader.

Equipment and Supplies:
- Computer or word processor
- Word processing software
- Draft paper
- Letterhead
- Printer
- Pen or pencil
- Highlighter
- Envelope
- Correspondence to be answered
- Other pertinent information needed to compose a letter
- Electronic or hard cover dictionary and thesaurus
- Writer's handbook
- Portfolio

Standards: Complete the procedure and all critical steps in _____ minutes with a minimum

score of _____ % within three attempts.

Scoring: Divide points earned by total possible points. Failure to perform a critical step that is indicated with an asterisk (*), will result in an unsatisfactory overall score.

Time began _____ **Time ended** _____

Steps	Possible Points	First Attempt	Second Attempt	Third Attempt
1. Read through any correspondence to be answered and highlight the specific questions that should be addressed.	10			
2. Make any necessary notes on the letter or a copy of the letter. A scrap sheet of paper may be used.	10			
3. Prepare a draft of the letter and save it in the computer or word processor, using good grammatical skills.	10			
4. Proofread a printed copy of the letter, using proofreader's marks to make corrections.	10			
5. Make any necessary corrections.	10			
6. Allow the physician or other interested party to proofread the letter, if the medical assistant is not the person whose signature will appear at the bottom.	10			

Steps	Possible Points	First Attempt	Second Attempt	Third Attempt
7. Make any final changes, then print the letter on stationery. Allow the person whose name appears at the bottom to sign the letter.	20	_____	_____	_____
8. Address the envelope using OCR guidelines and place the letter and any supporting documents inside.	10	_____	_____	_____
9. Mail the letter using correct postage.	10	_____	_____	_____

Comments:

Total Points Earned _____ Divided by _____ Total Possible Points = _____ % Score

Instructor's Signature _____

Procedure 12-2 Proofreading Written Correspondence

Task: To compose a clearly written, grammatically correct business letter, which is easily understandable by the reader, and to eliminate spelling errors.

Equipment and Supplies:
• Stationary
• Computer or typewriter
• Correspondence to be answered or notes

Standards: Complete the procedure and all critical steps in _____ minutes with a minimum

score of _____ % within three attempts.

Scoring: Divide points earned by total possible points. Failure to perform a critical step that is indicated with an asterisk (*), will result in an unsatisfactory overall score.

Time began _____ **Time ended** _____

Steps	Possible Points	First Attempt	Second Attempt	Third Attempt
1. Place the stationary into the printer or typewriter.	10			
2. Scan through the letter to be answered or the notes about the correspondence to be written and highlight any questions that should be answered or points to be made.	10			
3. Write the letter using grammatical guidelines.	10			
4. Print a draft copy of the letter. Read it carefully and highlight changes to be made or note any additions to be made. Use proofreaders' marks.	20			
5. Revise the letter using the notes.	10			
6. Read the letter once again on the screen. Complete a spell and grammatical check if those tools are available on the computer.	10			
7. Print a final draft. Read the letter word-for-word and check once again for errors.	10			
8. Have another person proofread especially important correspondence.	10			
9. Complete the final preparations for mailing the letter. Address the letter using guidelines for OCR and fast processing at the post office.	10			

Comments:

Total Points Earned _____ Divided by _____ Total Possible Points = _____ % Score

Instructor's Signature _____

Procedure 12-3 Preparing a FAX for Transmission

Task: To send a FAX from the medical office and assure that it arrives at its destination in a confidential manner.

Equipment and Supplies:
• FAX machine
• FAX cover sheet
• Correspondence to be sent

Standards: Complete the procedure and all critical steps in _____ minutes with a minimum score of _____ % within three attempts.

Scoring: Divide points earned by total possible points. Failure to perform a critical step that is indicated with an asterisk (*), will result in an unsatisfactory overall score.

Time began _____ **Time ended** _____

Steps	Possible Points	First Attempt	Second Attempt	Third Attempt
1. Fill out a FAX cover sheet. Include the name of the person sending the FAX, and the person's phone number. List the name of the person to receive the FAX and the FAX number where the document is being sent. Use cover sheets that contain a confidentiality statement.	20			
2. Note the number of pages that are being sent, including the cover page.	20			
3. Turn the last page upside down and write the fax number on the top of the document. Many machines require the documents to be in place prior to starting the fax. This allows the user to see the number without having to memorize it and make an error.	20			
4. Follow the instructions for individual FAX machines.	20			
5. Be sure the machine is set to provide a verification that the fax went through. Print the verification and attach it to the fax. Verify the arrival of critical FAX documents on the phone. File the fax and verification sheet in the appropriate location.	20			

Comments:

Total Points Earned _____ Divided by _____ Total Possible Points = _____ % Score

Instructor's Signature _____

Procedure 12-4 Opening the Daily Mail

Task: To sort through the mail that arrives in the medical office on a daily basis in an efficient way.

Equipment and Supplies:
- Computer or word processor
- Letterhead stationary
- Pen or pencil
- Highlighter
- Staple remover
- Paper clips
- Letter opener
- Date stamp
- Draft paper
- Stapler
- Transparent tape

Standards: Complete the procedure and all critical steps in _____ minutes with a minimum

score of _____ % within three attempts.

Scoring: Divide points earned by total possible points. Failure to perform a critical step that is indicated with an asterisk (*), will result in an unsatisfactory overall score.

Time began _____ **Time ended** _____

Steps	Possible Points	First Attempt	Second Attempt	Third Attempt
1. Sort the mail according to importance and urgency: • Physician's personal mail • Ordinary First Class mail • Checks from patients • Periodicals and newspapers • All other pieces, including drug samples	10			
2. Open the mail neatly and in an organized manner.	10			
3. Stack the envelopes so that they are all facing in the same direction.	10			
4. Pick up the top one and tap the envelope so that when you open it you will not cut the contents.	10			
5. Open all envelopes along the top edge for easiest removal of contents.	10			
6. Remove the contents of each envelope and hold the envelope to the light to see that nothing remains inside.	10			
7. Make a note of the postmark when this is important.	10			

Steps	Possible Points	First Attempt	Second Attempt	Third Attempt
8. Discard the envelope after you have checked to see that there is a return address on the message contained inside. Some offices make it a policy to attach the envelope to each piece of correspondence until it has received attention.	10			
9. Date stamp the letter and attach any enclosures.	10			
10. If there is an enclosure notation at the bottom of the letter, check to be certain that the enclosure was included. Should it be missing, indicate this on the notation by writing the word **no** and circling it.	10			

Comments:

Total Points Earned _____ Divided by _____ Total Possible Points = _____ % Score

Instructor's Signature _____

Procedure 12-5 Addressing Outgoing Mail Using U.S. Post Office OCR Guidelines

Task: To correctly address business correspondence so that the mail arrives and is processed by the U.S. Post Office as efficiently as possible.

Equipment and Supplies
- Envelopes
- Computer or typewriter
- Correspondence

Standards: Complete the procedure and all critical steps in _____ minutes with a minimum score of _____ % within three attempts.

Scoring: Divide points earned by total possible points. Failure to perform a critical step that is indicated with an asterisk (*), will result in an unsatisfactory overall score.

Time began _____ **Time ended** _____

Steps	Possible Points	First Attempt	Second Attempt	Third Attempt
1. Place the envelope into the printer or typewriter.	10			
2. Enter the word processing program, such as Microsoft Word, and check the "Tools" section for envelopes. If this is not available in the word processing program, or a typewriter is being used, judge the area on the envelope that can be read by the optical character reader (OCR). The address block should start no higher than 2¾ inches from the bottom. Leave a bottom margin of at least 5/8 inch and left and right margins of at least 1 inch. Nothing should be written or printed below the address block or to the right of it.	20			
3. Use dark type on a light background, no script or italics, and capitalize everything in the address.	10			
4. Type the address in block format, using only approved abbreviations and eliminating all punctuation.*	20			
5. Type the city, state, and zip code on the last line of the address.	10			
6. No line should have more than 27 total characters, including spaces.	10			

Steps	Possible Points	First Attempt	Second Attempt	Third Attempt
7. Leave a 5/8″ by 4¾″ space blank in the bottom right corner of the envelope.	**10**	_____	_____	_____
8. Mail addressed to other countries includes the city and postal code on the third line, and the name of the country on a fourth line.	**10**	_____	_____	_____

Comments:

Total Points Earned _____ Divided by _____ Total Possible Points = _____ % Score

Instructor's Signature _____

Procedure 13-1 Initiating a Medical File for a New Patient

Task: To initiate a medical file for a new patient that will contain all the personal data necessary for a complete medical record and any other information required by the agency.

Equipment and Supplies:
- Computer or typewriter
- Clerical supplies
- Information on filing system
- Registration form
- File Folder
- Label
- ID card for numeric system
- Cross-reference card
- Financial card
- Routing slip or encounter form
- Private conference area

Standards: Complete the procedure and all critical steps in _____ minutes with a minimum score of _____ % within three attempts.

Scoring: Divide points earned by total possible points. Failure to perform a critical step that is indicated with an asterisk (*), will result in an unsatisfactory overall score.

Time began _____ **Time ended** _____

Steps	Possible Points	First Attempt	Second Attempt	Third Attempt
1. Determine that the patient is new to the office.	10			
2. Obtain and record the required personal data.	10			
3. Type the information onto the patient history form.	10			
4. Review entire form.	10			
5. Select label and file folder for the record.	10			
6. Type the caption on the label and apply to folder	10			
7. For numeric filing, prepare a cross-reference.	10			
8. Prepare the financial card or enter into a computerized ledger.	10			
9. Place the patient's history and other required forms in the folder.	10			
10. Clip an encounter form or routing slip on the outside of the folder	10			

Comments:

Total Points Earned _____ Divided by _____ Total Possible Points = _____ % Score

Instructor's Signature _____

Procedure 13-2 Preparing an Informed Consent for Treatment Form

Task: To adequately and completely inform the patient regarding the treatment or procedure that he or she is to receive, and provide legal protection for the facility and the provider.

Equipment and Supplies:
• Pen
• Consent form

Standards: Complete the procedure and all critical steps in _____ minutes with a minimum

score of _____ % within three attempts.

Scoring: Divide points earned by total possible points. Failure to perform a critical step that is indicated with an asterisk (*), will result in an unsatisfactory overall score.

Time began _____ **Time ended** _____

Steps	Possible Points	First Attempt	Second Attempt	Third Attempt
1. After the physician provides the details of the procedure to be done, prepare the consent form. Be sure that the form addresses the following: a. the nature of the procedure or treatment b. the risks and/or benefits of the procedure or treatment c. any reasonable alternatives to the procedure or treatment d. the risks and/or benefits of each alternative e. the risks and/or benefits of not performing the procedure or treatment	20			
2. Personalize the form with the patient's name and any other demographic information that the form lists.	10			
3. Deliver the form to the physician for use as the patient is counseled about the procedure.	10			
4. Witness the signature of the patient on the form, if necessary. The physician will usually sign the form as well.	10			
5. Provide a copy of the consent form to the patient.	10			
6. Place the consent form in the patient's chart. The facility where the procedure is to be performed may require a copy.	10			

Steps	Possible Points	First Attempt	Second Attempt	Third Attempt
7. Ask the patient if he or she has any questions about the procedure. Refer questions that the medical assistant cannot or should not answer to the physician. Be sure that all of the questions expressed by the patient are answered.	20	_____	_____	_____
8. Provide information regarding the date and time for the procedure to the patient.	10	_____	_____	_____

Comments:

Total Points Earned _____ Divided by _____ Total Possible Points = _____ % Score

Instructor's Signature _____

Procedure 13-3 Adding Supplementary Items to Established Patient Files

Task: To initiate a medical file for a new patient that will contain all the personal data necessary for a complete medical record and any other information required by the agency.

Equipment and Supplies:
- Computer or typewriter
- Clerical supplies, sorter, stapler
- Information on filing system
- Mending tape
- Patient file folders
- Assorted correspondence and reports
- File stamp and a pen

Standards: Complete the procedure and all critical steps in _____ minutes with a minimum

score of _____ % within three attempts.

Scoring: Divide points earned by total possible points. Failure to perform a critical step that is indicated with an asterisk (*), will result in an unsatisfactory overall score.

Time began _____ **Time ended** _____

Steps	Possible Points	First Attempt	Second Attempt	Third Attempt
1. Group all papers according to patients' names.*	20			
2. Remove and pins or paper clips.	10			
3. Mend and damaged or torn records.	10			
4. Attach any small items to standard-sized paper.	10			
5. Staple any related papers together.	10			
6. Place your initials or FILE stamp in the upper left corner.	10			
7. Code the document by underlining or writing the patient's name in the upper right corner.	10			
8. Continue steps 2-7 until all documents have been conditioned, released, indexed, and coded.	10			
9. Place all documents in the sorter in filing sequence.	10			

Comments:

Total Points Earned _____ Divided by _____ Total Possible Points = _____ % Score

Instructor's Signature _____

Procedure 13-4 Preparing a Record Release Form

Task: To provide a legal document to another provider or healthcare facility that indicates the patient's consent to the release of his or her medical records.

Equipment and Supplies:
• Medical record release form
• Pen
• Envelope

Standards: Complete the procedure and all critical steps in _____ minutes with a minimum

score of _____ % within three attempts.

Scoring: Divide points earned by total possible points. Failure to perform a critical step that is indicated with an asterisk (*), will result in an unsatisfactory overall score.

Time began _____ **Time ended** _____

Steps	Possible Points	First Attempt	Second Attempt	Third Attempt
1. Explain to the patient that a medical record release form will be necessary to obtain records from another provider. If the patient is having records sent to another provider, a release will also be required.	20			
2. Review the record release form with the patient and ask if the form is understood or if there are any questions about the form.	20			
3. Have the patient sign the form in the space indicated. If other demographic information is required, such as a social security number or other names used, complete that information as well.	20			
4. Make a copy of the form for the file and then mail it to the appropriate facility. Note the date that the form was sent. Provide a copy to the patient if requested.	20			
5. Follow-up to assure that the requested records actually arrived.	20			

Comments:

Total Points Earned _____ Divided by _____ Total Possible Points = _____ % Score

Instructor's Signature _____

Student Name _____ Date _____ Score _____

Procedure 13-5 Transcribing a Machine-Dictated Letter Using a Computer or Word Processor

Task: To transcribe a machine-dictated letter into a mailable document without error or detectable corrections, using a computer or word processor.

Equipment and Supplies:
- Word processor, computer, or typewriter
- Transcribing machine
- Stationary
- Reference manual

Standards: Complete the procedure and all critical steps in _____ minutes with a minimum

score of _____ % within three attempts.

Scoring: Divide points earned by total possible points. Failure to perform a critical step that is indicated with an asterisk (*), will result in an unsatisfactory overall score.

Time began _____ Time ended _____

Steps	Possible Points	First Attempt	Second Attempt	Third Attempt
1. Assemble supplies.	10	_____	_____	_____
2. Set up the format for selected letter style.	20	_____	_____	_____
3. Keyboard the text while listening to the dictation.	20	_____	_____	_____
4. Edit the letter on the monitor.	20	_____	_____	_____
5. Execute a spell check.	20	_____	_____	_____
6. Direct the document to a printer.	10	_____	_____	_____

Comments:

Total Points Earned _____ Divided by _____ Total Possible Points = _____ % Score

Instructor's Signature _____

Procedure 13-6 Filing Medical Records and Documents Using the Alphabetical System

Task: To file records efficiently using an alphabetical system and assure that the records can be easily and quickly retrieved.

Equipment and Supplies:
- Medical records
- Physical filing equipment
- Cart to carry records, if needed
- Alphabetic file guide
- Staple remover
- Stapler
- Paper clips

Standards: Complete the procedure and all critical steps in _____ minutes with a minimum score of _____ % within three attempts.

Scoring: Divide points earned by total possible points. Failure to perform a critical step that is indicated with an asterisk (*), will result in an unsatisfactory overall score.

Time began _____ **Time ended** _____

Steps	Possible Points	First Attempt	Second Attempt	Third Attempt
1. Using alphabetical guidelines, place the records to be filed in alphabetical order. If a stack of documents is to be filed, place them in alphabetical order inside an alphabetic file guide or sorter. Use rules for filing documents alphabetically.	20	_____	_____	_____
2. Go to the filing storage equipment (shelves, cabinets, or drawers) and locate the spot in the alphabet for the first file.	20	_____	_____	_____
3. Place the file in the cabinet or drawer in correct alphabetical order.	20	_____	_____	_____
4. If adding a document to a file, place it on top, so that the most recent information is seen first. This puts the information in the file in reverse chronological order.	20	_____	_____	_____
5. Securely fasten documents to the chart. Do not just drop the documents inside the chart. Refile the chart in its proper place.	20	_____	_____	_____

Comments:

Total Points Earned _____ Divided by _____ Total Possible Points = _____ % Score

Instructor's Signature _____

Procedure 13-7 Filing Medical Records and Documents Using the Numeric System

Task: To file records efficiently using a numeric system and assure that the records can be easily and quickly retrieved.

Equipment and Supplies:
- Medical records
- Physical filing equipment
- Cart to carry records, if needed
- Numeric file guide
- Staple remover
- Stapler
- Paper clips

Standards: Complete the procedure and all critical steps in _____ minutes with a minimum

score of _____ % within three attempts.

Scoring: Divide points earned by total possible points. Failure to perform a critical step that is indicated with an asterisk (*), will result in an unsatisfactory overall score.

Time began _____ **Time ended** _____

Steps	Possible Points	First Attempt	Second Attempt	Third Attempt
1. Using numeric guidelines, place the records to be filed in numeric order. If a stack of documents is to be filed, write the chart number on the document. Use rules for filing documents alphabetically.	20	_____	_____	_____
2. Go to the filing storage equipment (shelves, cabinets, or drawers) and locate the numeric spot for the first file.	20	_____	_____	_____
3. Place the file in the cabinet or drawer in correct numeric order.	20	_____	_____	_____
4. If adding a document to a file, place it on top, so that the most recent information is seen first. This puts the information in the file in reverse chronological order.	20	_____	_____	_____
5. Securely fasten documents to the chart. Do not just drop the documents inside the chart.	20	_____	_____	_____

Comments:

Total Points Earned _____ Divided by _____ Total Possible Points = _____ % Score

Instructor's Signature _____

Procedure 13-8 Color Coding Patient Charts

Task: To color code patient charts using the agecy's established coding system to effectively facilitate filing and finding.

Equipment and Supplies:
- 20 Patient charts
- Information on filing system
- 20 file folders
- Full range of color labels

Standards: Complete the procedure and all critical steps in _____ minutes with a minimum score of _____ % within three attempts.

Scoring: Divide points earned by total possible points. Failure to perform a critical step that is indicated with an asterisk (*), will result in an unsatisfactory overall score.

Time began _____ **Time ended** _____

Steps	Possible Points	First Attempt	Second Attempt	Third Attempt
1. Assemble patient charts.	10			
2. Arrange charts in indexing order.	15			
3. Pick up the first chart and note the second letter of the surname.	15			
4. Chose a folder and/or caption label of the appropriate color.	15			
5. Type the patients' name on label in indexing order and apply to folder tab.	15			
6. Repeat steps 4 and 5 until all charts have been coded.	15			
7. Check any group for any isolated color.	15			

Comments:

Total Points Earned _____ Divided by _____ Total Possible Points = _____ % Score

Instructor's Signature _____

Procedure 14-1 Explaining Professional Fees

Task: To explain the physician's fees so that the patient understands his or her obligations and rights for privacy.

Equipment and Supplies:
• Patient's statement
• Copy of physician's fee schedule
• Quiet, private area with the patient feels free to ask questions

Standards: Complete the procedure and all critical steps in _____ minutes with a minimum

score of _____ % within three attempts.

Scoring: Divide points earned by total possible points. Failure to perform a critical step that is indicated with an asterisk (*), will result in an unsatisfactory overall score.

Time began _____ **Time ended** _____

Steps	Possible Points	First Attempt	Second Attempt	Third Attempt
1. Determine that the patient has the correct bill.	10	_____	_____	_____
2. Examine the bill for possible errors.	15	_____	_____	_____
3. Refer to the fee schedule for services rendered.	15	_____	_____	_____
4. Explain itemized billing: • Date of each service • Type of service rendered • Fee	15	_____	_____	_____
5. Display a professional attitude toward the patient.	15	_____	_____	_____
6. Determine whether the patient has specific concerns that may hinder payment.	15	_____	_____	_____
7. Make appropriate arrangements for a discussion between the physician and patient if further explanation is necessary for resolution of the problem.	15	_____	_____	_____

Comments:

Total Points Earned _____ Divided by _____ Total Possible Points = _____ % Score

Instructor's Signature _____

Procedure 14-2 Posting Service Charges and Payments Using Pegboard

Task: To post one day's charges and payments and computer the daily bookkeeping cycle using a pegboard.

Equipment and Supplies:
- Patient's statement
- Calculator
- Pen
- Daysheet
- Carbon
- Receipts
- Ledger cards
- Balances from previous day

Standards: Complete the procedure and all critical steps in _____ minutes with a minimum

score of _____ % within three attempts.

Scoring: Divide points earned by total possible points. Failure to perform a critical step that is indicated with an asterisk (*), will result in an unsatisfactory overall score.

Time began _____ **Time ended** _____

Steps	Possible Points	First Attempt	Second Attempt	Third Attempt
1. Prepare the board: • Place a new daysheet on the board. • Cover daysheet with carbon. • Place bank of receipts over the pegs, aligning the top receipt with the first open writing line on the daysheet.	5			
2. Carry forward balances from the previous day.	5			
3. Pull ledger cards for patient being seen today.	5			
4. Insert the ledger card under the first receipt, aligning the first available writing line of the card with the carbonized strip on the receipt.	5			
5. Enter the patientís name, the date, receipt number, and any existing balance from the ledger card.	5			
6. Detach the charge slip from the receipt and clip it to the patientís chart.	5			
7. Accept the returned charge slip at the end of the visit.	5			
8. Enter the appropriate fee from the fee schedule.	5			

Steps	Possible Points	First Attempt	Second Attempt	Third Attempt
9. Locate the receipt on the board with a number matching the charge slip.	5			
10. Reinsert the patientís ledger card under the receipt.	5			
11. Write the service code number and fee on the receipt.	5			
12. Accept the patient's payment and record the amount of payment and the new balance.	5			
13. Give the completed receipt to the patient.	5			
14. Follow your agency's procedure for refilling the ledger card.	5			
15. Repeat step 4 to 14 for each service of the day.	**10**			
16. Total all columns of the daysheet at the end of the day.	5			
17. Write preliminary totals in pencil.	5			
18. Complete proof of totals and enter totals in ink.	5			
19 Enter figures for accounts receivable control.	5			

Comments:

Total Points Earned _____ Divided by _____ Total Possible Points = _____ % Score

Instructor's Signature _____

Procedure 14-3 Making Credit Arrangements with a Patient

Task: To assist the patient in paying for services by making mutually beneficial credit arrangements according to established office policy.

Equipment and Supplies:
- Patient's ledger
- Calendar
- Truth in lending form
- Assignment of benefits form
- Patient's insurance form
- Private area for interview

Standards: Complete the procedure and all critical steps in _____ minutes with a minimum score of _____ % within three attempts.

Scoring: Divide points earned by total possible points. Failure to perform a critical step that is indicated with an asterisk (*), will result in an unsatisfactory overall score.

Time began _____ **Time ended** _____

Steps	Possible Points	First Attempt	Second Attempt	Third Attempt
1. Answer all questions about credit thoroughly and kindly.	10			
2. Inform the patient of the office policy regarding credit: • Payment at the time of first visit • Payment by bank card • Credit application	20			
3. Have the patient complete the credit application.	10			
4. Check the completed credit application.	10			
5. Discuss with the patient the possible arrangements and ask the patient to decide which of those arrangements is most suitable.	10			
6. Prepare the truth in lending form and have the patient sign it if the agreement requires more than four installments.	10			
7. Have the patient execute an assignment of insurance benefits.	10			
8. Make a copy of the patient's insurance ID and have the patient's sign a consent for release of the information to the insurance company.	10			
9. Keep credit information confidential.	10			

Comments:

Total Points Earned _____ Divided by _____ Total Possible Points = _____ % Score

Instructor's Signature _____

Student Name _____ Date _____ Score _____

Procedure 14-4 Preparing Monthly Billing Statements

Task: To Process monthly statements and evaluate accounts for collection procedures in accordance with the agency's credit policy.

Equipment and Supplies:
- Typewriter or computer
- Patient accounts
- Agency's credit policy
- Statement forms

Standards: Complete the procedure and all critical steps in _____ minutes with a minimum

score of _____ % within three attempts.

Scoring: Divide points earned by total possible points. Failure to perform a critical step that is indicated with an asterisk (*), will result in an unsatisfactory overall score.

Time began _____ **Time ended** _____

Steps	Possible Points	First Attempt	Second Attempt	Third Attempt
1. Assemble all accounts that have outstanding balances.	20			
2. Separate accounts that need special attention in accordance with the agency's credit policy.	20			
3. Prepare routine statements, including • Date the statement is prepared • Name and address of the person responsible for payment • Name of the patient, if different from the person responsible for payment • Itemization of dates, services, and charges for the month • Any unpaid balance carried forward (may or may not be itemized, depending on office policy)	20			
4. Determine the action to be taken on accounts separated in step 2.	20			
5. Make a note of the necessary action on the ledger card (telephone call, collection letter series, small claims court, or assignment of collection agency).	20			

Comments:

Total Points Earned _____ Divided by _____ Total Possible Points = _____ % Score

Instructor's Signature _____

Procedure 14-5 Aging Accounts Receivable

Task: To determine the age of accounts and decide what collection activity is needed.

Equipment and Supplies
- Patient ledger cards with a balance due
- Pen
- Computer
- Calculator

Standards: Complete the procedure and all critical steps in _____ minutes with a minimum

score of _____ % within three attempts.

Scoring: Divide points earned by total possible points. Failure to perform a critical step that is indicated with an asterisk (*), will result in an unsatisfactory overall score.

Time began _____ **Time ended** _____

Steps	Possible Points	First Attempt	Second Attempt	Third Attempt
1. Prompt the computer to compile a report on the age of accounts receivable. Many programs will have this report option that can be easily accessed.	10			
2. Divide the accounts into categories as listed below: • 0 to 30 days old • 30 to 60 days old • 60 to 90 days old • 90 to 120 days old • over 120 days old	20			
3. If the computer program does not perform this function, manually pull all ledger cards that have a balance due and divide them into the categories as listed above.	10			
4. Examine the accounts to see which are awaiting an insurance payment. Action need not be taken if an insurance payment is expected and is not long overdue. Return those ledgers to the ledger tray.	10			
5. Follow the office procedure for collections on the accounts left. Collection reminder stickers may be placed on the statements sent to the patient, or a collection letter may be sent. Be sure that the stickers are inside the envelope, not on the outside.	10			

Steps	Possible Points	First Attempt	Second Attempt	Third Attempt
6. Call patients whose accounts are over 90 days old. Attempt to make payment arrangements with the patient.	10			
7. Send a collection letter to patients whose accounts are over 120 days old, if indicated, to encourage the patient to pay the account. If it is the office policy, mention that the account is in danger of being sent to a collection agency.	10			
8. Add the total accounts receivable for each category and arrive at a figure outstanding for each. The physician may wish to have a report weekly or monthly on these figures.	10			
9. Note any arrangements made with patients regarding payment of the accounts in the chart and/or on the ledger. Send a follow-up letter to remind the patients of their payment agreements.	10			

Comments:

Total Points Earned _____ Divided by _____ Total Possible Points = _____ % Score

Instructor's Signature _____

Procedure 15-1 Assigning ICD-9-CM Codes

Task: To assign the proper ICD-9-CM code based on a medical documentation for auditing and billing purposes.

Equipment and Supplies:
- Patient medical record
- Current ICD-9-CM code book
- Medical dictionary

Standards: Complete the procedure and all critical steps in _____ minutes with a minimum

score of _____ % within three attempts.

Scoring: Divide points earned by total possible points. Failure to perform a critical step that is indicated with an asterisk (*), will result in an unsatisfactory overall score.

Time began _____ **Time ended** _____

Steps	Possible Points	First Attempt	Second Attempt	Third Attempt
1. Identify the key term in the diagnostic statement.	20			
2. Locate the diagnosis in the alphabetic index.	10			
3. Read and understand footnotes. NOTE: This includes any symbols, instructions, or cross-references.	10			
4. Locate the diagnosis in the Tabular List.	10			
5. Read and understand the inclusions and exclusions.	10			
6. Make certain you include 4th and 5th digits where available.	10			
7. Assign the code. NOTE: All diagnosis elements need to be identified. Double-check the code to insure an accurate transfer to the patient form.	30			

Comments:

Total Points Earned _____ Divided by _____ Total Possible Points = _____ % Score

Instructor's Signature _____

Procedure 16-1 Assigning CPT Codes

Task: To assign the proper CPT codes based on medical documentation for auditing and billing purposes.

Equipment and Supplies:
- Patient medical record
- Current CPT code book
- Medical dictionary

Standards: Complete the procedure and all critical steps in _____ minutes with a minimum score of _____ % within three attempts.

Scoring: Divide points earned by total possible points. Failure to perform a critical step that is indicated with an asterisk (*), will result in an unsatisfactory overall score.

Time began _____ **Time ended** _____

Steps	Possible Points	First Attempt	Second Attempt	Third Attempt
1. Identify if the patient is new or established. NOTE: An office (or outpatient) visit for the evaluation and management of a new patient requires these three key components: • A detailed history • A detailed examination • Medical decision-making of low complexity	10			
2. Indicate where the patient is being seen.	10			
3. Determine whether the visit is a consultation.	10			
4. Determine whether the visit is due to illness or is a preventative medical service.	10			
5. Determine the level of history.	10			
6. Determine the level of examination.	10			
7. Determine the level of medical decision making.	10			
8. Assign the most accurate CPT code.	30			

Comments:

Total Points Earned _____ Divided by _____ Total Possible Points = _____ % Score

Instructor's Signature _____

Procedure 17-1 Completing the Insurance Claim Form

Task: To accurately complete a CMS-1500 (formerly HCFA-1500) claim form.

Equipment and Supplies:
- Patient information form
- Photocopy of patient's insurance ID card
- Encounter Form
- Patient record
- Patient's ledger
- CMS-1500 form
- Typewriter or computer

Standards: Complete the procedure and all critical steps in _____ minutes with a minimum

score of _____ % within three attempts.

Scoring: Divide points earned by total possible points. Failure to perform a critical step that is indicated with an asterisk (*), will result in an unsatisfactory overall score.

Time began _____ **Time ended** _____

Steps	Possible Points	First Attempt	Second Attempt	Third Attempt
Patient/Insured Section				
Block 1 Check the type of health insurance coverage applicable to the claim.	2			
Block 1a Enter the patient's insurance identification number or Medicare ID number exactly as it appears on his/her insurance card.	2			
Block 2 Enter the patient's last name, first name and middle initial following OCR guidelines.	2			
Block 3 Enter the patient's birth date in MM DD YYYY format, and enter an "×" in the appropriate box for gender.	2			
Block 4 For commercial and Blue Cross/Blue Shield claims, enter "SAME" if patient and insured (policy-holder) are the same person. If the insured's name is different from the patient, enter the last name, first name, and middle initial in this block. If there is insurance primary to Medicare, list the name of the insured here. If Medicare is primary, leave blank. For CHAMPUS/TRICARE, enter the "sponsor's" name.	2			
Block 5 Enter the patient's street address on the first line, city and state on the second line, and the zip code and telephone number on the third line. Remember to use all capital letters and no punctuation.	2			

Steps	Possible Points	First Attempt	Second Attempt	Third Attempt
Block 6 Check the appropriate box for the patient's relationship to insured. If Medicare is primary, leave blank.	2			
Block 7 Enter the insured's address and telephone number, unless the insured and the patient are the same, in which case enter "SAME." Complete this item only when Blocks 4 and 11 are completed. For Medicare and Medicaid, leave blank.	2			
Block 8 Check the appropriate box for the patient's marital status and whether employed or a student.	2			
Block 9 (Required if 11d is marked "yes".) If the patient has other medical insurance coverage, and he/she is not the insured, enter the insured's name, and complete boxes 9a through 9d. If there is no other insurance, leave 9a through 9d blank and proceed to Block 10.	2			
Block 9a Enter the policy or group number of the insured's secondary insurance coverage. If the secondary policy is Medigap, enter the policy and/or group number preceded by **MEDIGAP.**	2			
Block 9b Enter the insured's birth date in MM DD YYYY format, and enter an "×" in the appropriate gender box.	2			
Block 9c Enter the name of the insured's employer or school, if applicable. Leave blank if a Medigap PayerID is entered in item 9d. Otherwise, enter the claims processing address of the Medigap insurer.	2			
Block 9d Enter the name of the secondary insurance plan or program. If the secondary insurer is a Medigap policy, enter the 9-digit PayerID number of the Medigap insurer. If there is no PayerID number, enter the Medigap insurance program or plan name.	2			
Block 10 Check the appropriate boxes in this section to identify whether the patient's condition was related to either his/her employment, auto accident, or other accident.	2			
Block 10a Check "no" unless the illness, accident, or injury was the result of employment or occurred on the job or in the process of performing one's job.	2			
Block 10b Check "no" unless the claim is due to an injury resulting from an automobile accident. In the case of an auto accident, enter the two-letter state code where the accident occurred.	2			

Steps	Possible Points	First Attempt	Second Attempt	Third Attempt
Block 10c Enter an "×" in the appropriate box.	2			
Block 10d This block is usually reserved for Medicaid as secondary payor claims. In some states, this block is used only if the patient is entitled to Medicaid. If this is the case, enter the patient's Medicaid number preceded by MCD. For Medicare, leave blank. Some third party payors want the word "attachment(s)" entered into this field if there are attachments included with the claim.	2			
Block 11 For commercial carriers, enter the group policy name/number from the patient's card. For BC/BS and Medicaid, leave blank. For insurance primary to Medicare, enter the insured's policy or group number. If Medicare is primary, the word "NONE" must appear in this block. By doing so indicates that Medicare is primary.	2			
NOTE: For a claim to be considered for Medicare Secondary Payer, a copy of the primary payer's explanation of benefits (EOB) must be included with the claim form.	2			
Block 11a Enter the insured's birth date and sex if different from Block 3. For Medicare and Medicaid, leave blank.	2			
Block 11b Enter the employer's name if applicable. On Medicare claims, if there is a second policy and the insured's status is retired, enter the date of retirement preceded by the word "RETIRED."	2			
Block 11c Enter the 9-digit Payer ID number of the primary insurer. If no such number exists, enter the complete name of the primary payer's program or plan name.	2			
Block 11d Check "no" if patient is covered by only one insurance policy. If the answer is "yes," give the name of the company and any other information available in Block 9. For Medicare and Medicaid, leave blank.	2			
Block 12 The patient or authorized person must sign and date this item unless a signature is on file. If this is the case, the words "SIGNATURE ON FILE" should be entered here. Leave blank on Medicaid claims.	2			
Block 13 The patient or authorized person should sign and date this item if he or she agrees that benefits are to be paid directly to the provider. For Medicare supplements and cross-over claims, "SIGNATURE ON FILE" must also appear in this block. For Medicaid, leave blank.	2			

Steps	Possible Points	First Attempt	Second Attempt	Third Attempt

Physician/Supplier Information

Block 14   Enter the date of the first symptom of the current illness, injury, or pregnancy in this block if one is documented in the chart notes or the date of the last menstrual cycle if the claim is related to pregnancy.

	2			

Block 15   Enter the date the patient was first treated for this condition. Leave blank for Medicare claims.

	2			

Block 16   Enter date(s) patient unable to work in current occupation if it is a workers' compensation claim. Not required for most other carriers.

	2			

Block 17   Enter the name of the referring (or ordering) physician, if applicable.

	2			

Block 17a   Enter the UPIN/NPI number of the referring/ordering physician listed in Block 17.

	2			

Block 18   If the claim is for a related hospital stay, enter the dates of hospital admission and discharge. If the patient has not been discharged, leave the "to" box blank.

	2			

Block 19   This block is usually left blank. Some private payors insert the word "attachment(s)" when specific documentation accompanies the claim.

	2			

Block 20   If laboratory procedures are listed on the claim in Block 24, and these services were performed in the provider's facility, the "NO" box in is checked with an "×" or left blank. If lab work shown on the claim was done by an outside lab and billed to the provider, check the "YES" box, and enter the total amount of the charges. Leave this block blank if no lab tests were done.

	2			

Block 21   Enter the patient's diagnosis(es) using ICD-9-CM code number(s), listing the primary diagnosis first. Up to four codes (in priority order) can be entered in Block 21.

	2			

Block 22   Required only for replacement claims for Medicaid. Enter the appropriate 3-digit replacement code followed by the 17-digit transaction control number of the most current incorrectly paid claim.

	2			

Block 23   For private and commercial carriers and Medicaid, enter the 10-digit prior authorization number for those procedures requiring prior approval assigned by the peer review organization (PRO). Consult the specific guidelines for the payor to whom the claim is being submitted.

	2			

Steps	Possible Points	First Attempt	Second Attempt	Third Attempt
Block 24a The first date of service for the charge on this line should be placed in the "From" column. When a claim is for more than one day of the same service on a line item, the days must be in consecutive order. The last date of service is required in the "To" column. Enter the month, day, and year (in the MM DD YYYY format) for each procedure, service, or supply. When "from" and "to" dates are shown for a series of identical services, enter the number of days or units in 24G.	2			
Block 24b Enter the appropriate place of service code.	2			
Block 24c Enter the appropriate type of service code. NOTE: For private payors and Medicare, leave blank. All others, refer to specific guidelines.	2			
Block 24d Enter the procedure, service, or supply code using appropriate 5-digit CPT or HCPCS procedure code. Enter a two-position modifier when applicable.	2			
Block 24e Link the procedure/service code back to the diagnosis code in Block 21 by indicating the applicable number of the diagnosis code (1, 2, 3 or 4) to that line's procedure code.	2			
Block 24f Enter the charge for each listed procedure, supply, and /or service.	2			
Block 24g Enter the number of days or units. If only one service is performed, enter the number 1.	2			
Block 24h Leave blank for all claims with the exception of certain Medicaid claims.	2			
Block 24i For certain carriers, enter an "X" or "E" as appropriate if documentation indicates a medical emergency existed. Leave blank for Medicare claims.	2			
Block 24j For commercial claims, BC/BS, Medicare, Medicaid, and TRICARE, leave blank. (Refer to specific third-payor guidelines.)	2			
Block 24k Enter the five-digit number that has been assigned when the provider was approved by the third-party payor. For Medicare, it is referred to as the "billing number." Blue Cross-Blue Shield and Medicaid have their own numbers. This is not the same of the UPIN number.	2			
Block 25 Enter the provider's nine-digit Federal tax identification number and check the appropriate box in this field; or, in the case of an unincorporated practice or sole proprietorship, enter the provider's social security number.	2			

Steps	Possible Points	First Attempt	Second Attempt	Third Attempt
Block 26 Enter the patient's account number as assigned by the supplier's accounting system, if available. If you are submitting the claim electronically, you are required to provide a patient account number.	2			
Block 27 Check the appropriate block to indicate whether the provider accepts assignment of benefits. If the supplier is a *participating provider* (PAR), assignment must be accepted for all covered charges. For nonPAR provider's, this can be left blank. For Medicaid, check "YES."	2			
Block 28 Total column 24f and enter the total charges in this field.	2			
Block 29 Enter the total amount, if any, that has been paid by the patient. Leave blank if no payment has been made.	2			
Block 30 Used when there is a secondary insurance. Enter the balance owing as indicated on the explanation of benefits (EOB).	2			
Block 31 Enter the signature of the provider, or his/her representative and his or her initials, and the date the form was signed. The signature may be typed, stamped, or handwritten; however, the characters should not fall outside of the block.	2			
Block 32 Enter the name and address of the facility where the services were performed if other than patient's home or physician's office. For Medicare, enter the name and address of the facility regardless of where services were provided.	2			
Block 33 Enter the provider's billing name, address, zip code, and telephone number. Also, enter the billing number (from Block 24k). Enter the Group NPI number, if the provider is a member of a group practice. Refer to specific third-payor guidelines.	2			

Comments:

Total Points Earned _____ Divided by _____ Total Possible Points = _____ % Score

Instructor's Signature _____

Procedure 18-1 Obtaining a Managed Care Precertification

Task: Using the information in the case study, obtain precertification from a patient's HMO for requested services/procedures.

Equipment and Supplies:
- Patient record
- Precertification form
- Patient's insurance information
- Telephone/FAX machine
- Pen/Pencil

Standards: Complete the procedure and all critical steps in _____ minutes with a minimum

score of _____ % within three attempts.

Scoring: Divide points earned by total possible points. Failure to perform a critical step that is indicated with an asterisk (*), will result in an unsatisfactory overall score.

Time began _____ **Time ended** _____

Steps	Possible Points	First Attempt	Second Attempt	Third Attempt
1. Assemble the necessary documents and equipment.	20			
2. Examine the patient record, and determine the service/procedure for which preauthorization is being requested, including the specialist's name and phone number, and the reason for the request.	20			
3. Complete the referral form, providing all pertinent information requested.	20			
4. Proofread the completed form to ascertain accuracy.	20			
5. Role play the act of faxing the completed form to the patient's insurance carrier. Place a copy of the completed form in the patient's medical record.	20			

Documentation in the Medical Record

_____
_____
_____
_____

Comments:

Total Points Earned _____ Divided by _____ Total Possible Points = _____ % Score

Instructor's Signature _____

Procedure 18-2 Obtaining a Managed Care Referral

Task: Using the information in the case study, accurately complete a referral form for the managed care patient.

Equipment and Supplies:
- Patient record
- Referral form
- Patient's insurance information
- Pen/Pencil

Standards: Complete the procedure and all critical steps in _____ minutes with a minimum

score of _____ % within three attempts.

Scoring: Divide points earned by total possible points. Failure to perform a critical step that is indicated with an asterisk (*), will result in an unsatisfactory overall score.

Time began _____ **Time ended** _____

Steps	Possible Points	First Attempt	Second Attempt	Third Attempt
1. Assemble the necessary documents and equipment.	20			
2. Examine the patient record, and determine the service for which the patient is to be referred, including the specialist's name and phone number, and the reason for the referral.	20			
3. Role plan with a partner the act of telephoning the patient's insurance carrier.	20			
4. Complete the referral form, providing all information requested.	20			
5. Proofread the completed form to ascertain accuracy. Place a copy of the completed form in the patient's medical record.	20			

Documentation in the Medical Record

_____

_____

_____

_____

Comments:

Total Points Earned _____ Divided by _____ Total Possible Points = _____ % Score

Instructor's Signature _____

Student Name _____ Date _____ Score _____

Procedure 19-1 Writing Checks in Payment of Bills

Task: To correctly write checks for payment of bills.

Equipment and Supplies:
- Checkbook
- Bills to be paid

Standards: Complete the procedure and all critical steps in _____ minutes with a minimum

score of _____ % within three attempts.

Scoring: Divide points earned by total possible points. Failure to perform a critical step that is indicated with an asterisk (*), will result in an unsatisfactory overall score.

Time began _____ **Time ended** _____

Steps	Possible Points	First Attempt	Second Attempt	Third Attempt
1. Locate bill to be paid. Fill out stub first.	10			
2. Complete check and stub with pen or typewriter.	10			
3. Date the check.	10			
4. Write the Payee on the appropriate line.	10			
5. Leave no space before the name and follow with three dashes. Omit personal titles.	10			
6. Enter amount correctly and in a manner that prevents alteration.*	20			
7. Verify amount with check stub.	20			
8. Make a notation on the bill that is being paid. Include date and check number. File.	10			

Comments:

Total Points Earned _____ Divided by _____ Total Possible Points = _____ % Score

Instructor's Signature _____

Procedure 19-2 Preparing a Bank Deposit

Task: To prepare a bank deposit for the day's receipts and complete appropriate office records related to the deposit.

Equipment and Supplies:
- Currency
- Six checks for deposit
- Deposit slip
- Endorsement stamp (optional)
- Typewriter
- Envelope

Standards: Complete the procedure and all critical steps in _____ minutes with a minimum

score of _____ % within three attempts.

Scoring: Divide points earned by total possible points. Failure to perform a critical step that is indicated with an asterisk (*), will result in an unsatisfactory overall score.

Time began _____ **Time ended** _____

Steps	Possible Points	First Attempt	Second Attempt	Third Attempt
1. Organize currency.	10			
2. Total the currency and record the amount on the deposit slip.	10			
3. Place restrictive endorsement on checks.*	20			
4. List each check separately on the deposit slip by ABA number or patient last name.	20			
5. Total the amount of currency and checks and enter on deposit slip.	10			
6. Enter the amount of the deposit in the checkbook.	10			
7. Keep a copy of the deposit slip for office records.	10			
8. Place currency, checks, and deposit in envelope for transport to bank.	10			

Comments:

Total Points Earned _____ Divided by _____ Total Possible Points = _____ % Score

Instructor's Signature _____

Procedure 19-3 Reconciling a Bank Statement

Task: To reconcile a bank statement with checking account.

Equipment and Supplies:
- Ending balance of previous statement
- Current bank statement
- Cancelled checks for current month
- Checkbook stubs
- Calculator
- Pen

Standards: Complete the procedure and all critical steps in _____ minutes with a minimum

score of _____ % within three attempts.

Scoring: Divide points earned by total possible points. Failure to perform a critical step that is indicated with an asterisk (*), will result in an unsatisfactory overall score.

Time began _____ **Time ended** _____

Steps	Possible Points	First Attempt	Second Attempt	Third Attempt
1. Compare opening balance of the new statement with the closing balance of previous statement.	10			
2. Compare canceled checks with items on statement.	10			
3. Arrange checks in numerical order and compare to stubs.	10			
4. Place a checkmark on the matching stub.	10			
5. List and total outstanding checks.	10			
6. Verify that all previous outstanding checks have cleared.	10			
7. Subtract the total of outstanding checks from the statement balance.*	10			
8. Add to the total in Step 7 any deposits made but not included in statement balance.	10			
9. Total any bank charges that appear on the bank statement and subtract them from the checkbook balance.	10			
10. If the checkbook and statement do not agree, match bank statement entries with the checkbook entries.	10			

Comments:

Total Points Earned _____ Divided by _____ Total Possible Points = _____ % Score

Instructor's Signature _____

Student Name _____ Date _____ Score _____

Procedure 20-1 Making Travel Arrangements

Task: To make travel arrangements for the physician or another staff member.

Equipment and Supplies:
- Travel plan
- Telephone
- Telephone directory
- Typewriter or computer
- Typing paper

Standards: Complete the procedure and all critical steps in _____ minutes with a minimum score of _____ % within three attempts.

Scoring: Divide points earned by total possible points. Failure to perform a critical step that is indicated with an asterisk (*), will result in an unsatisfactory overall score.

Time began _____ **Time ended** _____

Steps	Possible Points	First Attempt	Second Attempt	Third Attempt
1. Verify the dates of the planned trip. • Desired date and time of departure • Desired date and time of return • Preferred mode of transportation • Number in party • Preferred lodging and price range • Preferred ticketing method (electronic or paper)	20	_____	_____	_____
2. Telephone a trusted travel agency to arrange for transportation and lodging reservations.	10	_____	_____	_____
3. Arrange for traveler's checks, if desired.	10	_____	_____	_____
4. Pick up tickets/e-receipts or arrange for delivery	10	_____	_____	_____
5. Check tickets to confirm conformance with the travel plan	10	_____	_____	_____
6. Check to see that hotel and air reservations are confirmed.	10	_____	_____	_____
7. Prepare an itinerary, including all the necessary information • Date and time of departure • Flight numbers or identifying information of other modes of travel • Mode of transportation to hotel(s) • Name, address, and telephone number of hotel(s), with confirmation numbers if available • Name, address, and telephone number of travel agency • Date and time of return	10	_____	_____	_____

Steps	Possible Points	First Attempt	Second Attempt	Third Attempt
8. Place one copy of itinerary in the office file.	10	_____	_____	_____
9. Give several copies of the itinerary to the traveler.	10	_____	_____	_____

Comments:

Total Points Earned _____ Divided by _____ Total Possible Points = _____ % Score

Instructor's Signature _____

Procedure 20-2 Arranging a Group Meeting

Task: To plan and execute a productive meeting that will result in achieved goals.

Equipment and Supplies:
- Meeting room
- Agenda
- Visual aids and equipment
- Handouts
- Stopwatch or clock
- Computer or word processor
- Paper
- List of items for the agenda

Standards: Complete the procedure and all critical steps in _____ minutes with a minimum

score of _____ % within three attempts.

Scoring: Divide points earned by total possible points. Failure to perform a critical step that is indicated with an asterisk (*), will result in an unsatisfactory overall score.

Time began _____ **Time ended** _____

Steps	Possible Points	First Attempt	Second Attempt	Third Attempt
1. Determine the purpose of the meeting and draft a list of the items to be discussed. Include the desired results of the meeting.	10			
2. Determine where the meeting will be held, the time and date of the meeting, and the individuals who should attend.	10			
3. Send a memo, email, or letter to the individuals who should attend the meeting at least ten days in advance, if possible. Send a copy to any supervisors who should be kept informed about the issues to be raised in the meeting.	10			
4. Be sure that the notice includes the following information: a. date b. time c. place d. directions, if not in a common meeting room or away from the office e. speakers and/or meeting topics f. cost and registration information, if applicable g. list of items individuals should bring to the meeting	10			
5. Finalize the list of items to discuss and place them in priority order.	10			

Steps	Possible Points	First Attempt	Second Attempt	Third Attempt
6. Delegate any tasks that others can accomplish and follow-up to be sure that they fulfill their duties prior to the meeting.	10			
7. Assign a staff member the task of keeping notes and keeping time during the meeting.	10			
8. Make a list of all items that need to be taken to the meeting, including equipment such as microphones, projectors, screens, computers, disks containing presentations, etc.	10			
9. Compile the final agenda for the meeting.	10			
10. On the meeting day, transport all items needed to the meeting room. Begin and end the meeting on time. Stay on track and follow the agenda.	10			

Comments:

Total Points Earned _____ Divided by _____ Total Possible Points = _____ % Score

Instructor's Signature _____

Student Name _____ Date _____ Score _____

Procedure 23-1 Accounting for Petty Cash

Task: To establish a petty cash fund, maintain an accurate record of expenditures for 1 month, and replenish the fund as necessary.

Equipment and Supplies:
- Form for petty cash fund
- Pad of vouchers
- Disbursement journal
- Two checks
- List of petty cash expenditures

Standards: Complete the procedure and all critical steps in _____ minutes with a minimum

score of _____ % within three attempts.

Scoring: Divide points earned by total possible points. Failure to perform a critical step that is indicated with an asterisk (*), will result in an unsatisfactory overall score.

Time began _____ **Time ended** _____

Steps	Possible Points	First Attempt	Second Attempt	Third Attempt
1. Determine the amount needed in the petty cash fund.	10			
2. Write a check in the determined amount.	10			
3. Record the beginning balance in the petty cash fund.	10			
4. Post the amount to miscellaneous on the disbursement record.	10			
5. Prepare a petty cash voucher for each amount withdrawn from the fund.	10			
6. Record each voucher in the petty cash record and enter the new balance.	10			
7. Write a check to replenish the fund as necessary. NOTE: The total of the vouchers plus the fund balance must equal the beginning amount.	10			
8. Total the expense columns and post to the appropriate accounts in the disbursement record.	10			
9. Record the amount added to the fund.	10			
10. Record the new balance in the petty cash fund.	10			

Documentation in the Medical Record

_____

_____

_____

_____

Comments:

Total Points Earned _____ Divided by _____ Total Possible Points = _____ % Score

Instructor's Signature _____

Procedure 23-2 Processing an Employee Payroll

Task: To process payroll and compensate employees, making deductions accurately.

Equipment and Supplies:
• Checkbook
• Computer and payroll software, if applicable
• Pen
• Tax withholding tables
• Federal employers tax guide

Standards: Complete the procedure and all critical steps in _____ minutes with a minimum

score of _____ % within three attempts.

Scoring: Divide points earned by total possible points. Failure to perform a critical step that is indicated with an asterisk (*), will result in an unsatisfactory overall score.

Time began _____ **Time ended** _____

Steps	Possible Points	First Attempt	Second Attempt	Third Attempt
1. Be sure that all information has been collected on the employees, including a copy of the social security card, a W-4 form, and an I-9 form.	20			
2. Review the time cards for all employees. Determine if any employees need counseling due to late arrivals or habitual absences.	20			
3. Figure the salary or hourly wages that are due the employee for the period worked.	20			
4. Figure the deductions that must be taken from the paycheck. This usually includes, but is not limited to: • Federal, state, and local taxes • Social security withholdings • Medicare withholdings • Other deductions, such as insurance, savings, etc. • Donations to organizations, such as the United Way	20			
5. Write the check for the balance due the employee. Most software programs can print the checks and explanations of deductions.	20			

Comments:

Total Points Earned _____ Divided by _____ Total Possible Points = _____ % Score

Instructor's Signature _____

Procedure 23-3 Establishing and Maintaining a Supply Inventory and Ordering System

Task: To establish an inventory of all expendable supplies in the physician's office and follow an efficient plan of order control using a card system.

Equipment and Supplies:
- File box
- Inventory and order control cards
- List of supplies on hand
- Metal tabs
- Reorder tabs
- Pen or pencil

Standards: Complete the procedure and all critical steps in _____ minutes with a minimum

score of _____ % within three attempts.

Scoring: Divide points earned by total possible points. Failure to perform a critical step that is indicated with an asterisk (*), will result in an unsatisfactory overall score.

Time began _____ **Time ended** _____

Steps	Possible Points	First Attempt	Second Attempt	Third Attempt
1. Write the name of each item on a separate card.	10			
2. Write the amount of each item on hand in the space provided.	10			
3. Place a reorder tag at the point where the supply should be replenished.	20			
4. Place a metal tab over the *order* section of the card.	20			
5. When the order has been placed, note the date and quantity ordered and move the table to the *on order* section of the card.	20			
6. Then the order is received, note the date and quantity in the appropriate column, remove the tab, and refile the card. NOTE: If the order is only partially filled, let the tab remain until the order is complete.	20			

Comments:

Total Points Earned _____ Divided by _____ Total Possible Points = _____ % Score

Instructor's Signature _____

Procedure 23-4 Preparing a Purchase Order

Task: To prepare an accurate purchase order for supplies or equipment.

Equipment and Supplies:
• List of current inventory
• Purchase order
• Pen
• Phone
• Fax machine

Standards: Complete the procedure and all critical steps in _____ minutes with a minimum

score of _____ % within three attempts.

Scoring: Divide points earned by total possible points. Failure to perform a critical step that is indicated with an asterisk (*), will result in an unsatisfactory overall score.

Time began _____ **Time ended** _____

Steps	Possible Points	First Attempt	Second Attempt	Third Attempt
1. Review the current inventory and determine what items need to be ordered.	10			
2. Complete the purchase order accurately, filling in all applicable spaces and blanks with the information requested.	15			
3. List the items to be ordered, including quantity, item numbers, size, color, price, and extended price. Be sure that all applicable information is included.	15			
4. Provide the physician's signature, DEA certificate, and medical license where needed.	15			
5. Call in, fax, mail, or submit the order electronically to the vendor. Keep a copy for your records. Keep any verification provided that the order was received.	15			
6. Note on the inventory which items are on order.	15			
7. Keep a copy of the order in the appropriate place in the office filing system.	15			

Comments:

Total Points Earned _____ Divided by _____ Total Possible Points = _____ % Score

Instructor's Signature _____

Procedure 24-1 Using an Automated External Defibrillator (AED)

Task: To defibrillate adult victims with cardiac arrest.

Equipment and Supplies:
- Practice AED
- Approved mannequin

Standards: Complete the procedure and all critical steps in _____ minutes with a minimum

score of _____ % within three attempts.

Scoring: Divide points earned by total possible points. Failure to perform a critical step that is indicated with an asterisk (*), will result in an unsatisfactory overall score.

Time began _____ **Time ended** _____

Steps	Possible Points	First Attempt	Second Attempt	Third Attempt
1. Place the AED near the victim's left ear. Turn the AED on.	20			
2. Attach electrode pads as pictured on the AED electrodes at the sternum and apex of the heart. Make sure pads have complete contact with the victim's chest and they do not overlap.	20			
3. All rescuers must clear away from the victim. Press the ANALYZE button. The AED will analyze the victim's coronary status, will announce if the victim is going to be shocked, and automatically charges the electrodes.	20			
4. All rescuers must clear away from the victim.* Press the SHOCK button if the machine is not automated. May repeat 1 to 2 more analyze-shock cycles.	20*			
5. If the machine gives the "no shock indicated" signal, assess the victim. Check the carotid pulse and breathing status and keep the AED attached until EMS arrives.	20			

Documentation in the Medical Record

_____

_____

_____

_____

Comments:

Total Points Earned _____ Divided by _____ Total Possible Points = _____ % Score

Instructor's Signature _____

Student Name _____ Date _____ Score _____

Procedure 24-2 Responding to a Patient with an Obstructed Airway

Task: To remove an airway obstruction and restore ventilation.

Equipment and Supplies:
• Nonsterile gloves
• Ventilation mask (for unconscious victim)
• Approved mannequin to practice unconscious Foreign Body Airway Obstruction (FBAO).

Standards: Complete the procedure and all critical steps in _____ minutes with a minimum

score of _____ % within three attempts.

Scoring: Divide points earned by total possible points. Failure to perform a critical step that is indicated with an asterisk (*), will result in an unsatisfactory overall score.

Time began _____ **Time ended** _____

Steps	Possible Points	First Attempt	Second Attempt	Third Attempt
1. Ask, "Are you choking?" If victim indicates yes, ask "Can you speak?". If unable to speak, tell the victim you are going to help.*	10			
2. Stand behind the victim with feet slightly apart.	5			
3. Reach around the victim's abdomen and place an index finger into the victim's navel or at the level of the belt buckle. Make a fist of the opposite hand (do not tuck the thumb into the fist) and place the thumb side of the fist against the victim's abdomen above the navel. If the victim is pregnant, place the fist above the enlarged uterus. If the victim is obese, it may be necessary to place the fist higher in the abdomen. It may be necessary to perform chest thrusts on a victim who is pregnant or obese.	5			
4. Place the opposite hand over the fist and give abdominal thrusts in a quick upward movement.	5			
5. Repeat the abdominal thrusts until the object is expelled or the victim becomes unresponsive.	5			
Unresponsive Victim				
6. Activate the emergency response system.*	10			
7. Put on gloves if available and get ventilation mask. Open the victim's mouth and perform a finger sweep to determine if the foreign object is in the mouth and to remove it.	5			

Copyright © 2003, Elsevier Science (USA). All rights reserved. 253

Steps	Possible Points	First Attempt	Second Attempt	Third Attempt
8. Open the airway with a head-tilt, jaw-thrust maneuver and attempt to ventilate with 2 slow breaths. If breaths do not go in (chest does not rise), retilt the head and try to ventilate again.	5			
9. If ventilation is unsuccessful, move to the victim's feet and kneel across the victim's thighs. Place the heel of one hand above the navel but below the xiphoid process of the sternum. Place the other hand on top of the first, with the fingers elevated off of the abdomen. Administer 5 abdominal thrusts.	5			
10. Move back beside the head of the victim and repeat the finger sweep. If the obstruction is not found, continue cycles of 2 rescue breaths, 5 abdominal thrusts, and finger sweep until either the obstruction is removed or EMS arrives.	5			
11. If the obstruction is removed, assess the victim for breathing and circulation. If a pulse is present, but no breathing, begin rescues breathing. If there is no pulse, begin CPR.	5			
12. Once patient is either stabilized or EMS has taken over care, remove gloves and the ventilator mask valve and dispose in the biohazard container. Disinfect the ventilator mask per manufacturer recommendations. Wash hands.	5			
13. Document the procedure and patient condition.	5			

Documentation in the Medical Record

_____

_____

_____

_____

Comments:

Total Points Earned _____ Divided by _____ Total Possible Points = _____ % Score

Instructor's Signature _____

Procedure 24-3 Administering Oxygen

Task: To provide oxygen for a patient in respiratory distress.

Equipment and Supplies:
- Portable oxygen tank
- Pressure regulator
- Flow meter
- Nasal cannula with connecting tubing

Standards: Complete the procedure and all critical steps in _____ minutes with a minimum

score of _____ % within three attempts.

Scoring: Divide points earned by total possible points. Failure to perform a critical step that is indicated with an asterisk (*), will result in an unsatisfactory overall score.

Time began _____ **Time ended** _____

Steps	Possible Points	First Attempt	Second Attempt	Third Attempt
1. Gather equipment and wash hands.	10			
2. Identify the patient and explain the procedure.	10			
3. Check the pressure gauge on the tank to determine the amount of oxygen in the tank.	10			
4. If necessary, open the cylinder on the tank one full counterclockwise turn and attach the cannula tubing to the flowmeter.	20			
5. Adjust the administration of the oxygen according to the physician's order. Check to make sure the oxygen is flowing through the cannula.	10			
6. Insert the cannula tips into the nostrils and adjust the tubing around the back of the patient's ears.	10			
7. Make sure the patient is comfortable and answer any questions.	10			
8. Wash hands.	10			
9. Document the procedure including the number of liters of oxygen being administered and the patient's condition. Continue to monitor the patient throughout the procedure and document any changes in condition.	10			

Documentation in the Medical Record

_____

_____

_____

_____

Comments:

Total Points Earned _____ Divided by _____ Total Possible Points = _____ % Score

Instructor's Signature _____

Procedure 24-4 Providing Rescue Breathing and Performing One Man CPR

Task: To restore a victim's breathing and blood circulation when respiration and pulse stop.

Equipment and Supplies:
• Nonsterile gloves
• CPR ventilator mask
• Approved mannequin

Standards: Complete the procedure and all critical steps in _____ minutes with a minimum

score of _____ % within three attempts.

Scoring: Divide points earned by total possible points. Failure to perform a critical step that is indicated with an asterisk (*), will result in an unsatisfactory overall score.

Time began _____ **Time ended** _____

Steps	Possible Points	First Attempt	Second Attempt	Third Attempt
1. Establish unresponsiveness. Tap the victim and ask, Are you OK? Wait for victim to respond.	10			
2. Activate the emergency response system. Put on gloves and get ventilator mask.	5			
3. Tilt the victim's head and lift the chin. Look, listen, and feel for signs of breathing. Place your ear over the mouth and listen for breathing. Watch the rising and falling of the chest for evidence of breathing.	10			
4. If breathing is absent or inadequate, place the ventilator mask over the victim's mouth and give 2 slow breaths (2 seconds per breath), holding the ventilator mask tightly against the face while tilting the victim's chin back to open the airway. Allow time for exhalation between breaths.	10			
5. Check the carotid pulse. If a pulse is present, continue rescue breathing (1 breath every 5 seconds, about 10 to 12 breaths per minute). If no signs of circulation are present, begin cycles of 15 chest compressions (at a rate of about 100 compressions per minute) followed by 2 slow breaths.	10			
6. Kneel at the victim's side opposite the chest. Move your fingers up the ribs to the point where the sternum and the ribs join. Your middle fingers should fit into the area and your index finger should be next to it across the sternum.	10			

Steps		Possible Points	First Attempt	Second Attempt	Third Attempt
7.	Place the heel of your hand on the chest midline over the sternum, just above your index finger.	5			
8.	Place your other hand on top of your first hand and lift your fingers upward off of the chest.	5			
9.	Bring your shoulders directly over the victim's sternum as you compress downward, and keep your arms straight.	5			
10.	Depress the sternum $1\frac{1}{2}$ to 2 inches for an adult victim. Relax the pressure on the sternum after each compression but do not remove your hands from the victim's sternum.	10			
11.	After performing 15 compressions (at a rate of about 100 compressions per minute), open the airway and give 2 slow breaths.	5			
12.	After 4 cycles of compressions and breaths (15:2 ratio, about 1 minute) recheck breathing and carotid pulse. If there is a pulse but no breathing, continue rescue breathing (1 breath every 5 seconds, about 10 to 12 breaths per minute) and reevaluate the victim's breathing and pulse every few minutes. If there are no signs of circulation, continue 15:2 cycles of compressions and ventilations, starting with chest compressions. Continue giving CPR until the EMS relieves you.	5			
13.	Remove gloves and the ventilator mask valve and dispose in the biohazard container. Disinfect the ventilator mask per manufacturer recommendations. Wash hands.	5			
14.	Document the procedure and patient condition.	5			

Documentation in the Medical Record

_____

_____

_____

_____

Comments:

Total Points Earned _____ Divided by _____ Total Possible Points = _____ % Score

Instructor's Signature _____

Procedure 24-5 Caring for a Patient who Fainted

Task: To provide emergency care and assessment of a patient who has fainted.

Equipment and Supplies:
- Sphygmomanometer
- Stethoscope
- Watch with second hand
- Blanket
- Foot stool or box
- Physician may order oxygen:
  - Portable oxygen tank
  - Pressure regulator
  - Flow meter
  - Nasal cannula with connecting tubing

Standards: Complete the procedure and all critical steps in _____ minutes with a minimum

score of _____ % within three attempts.

Scoring: Divide points earned by total possible points. Failure to perform a critical step that is indicated with an asterisk (*), will result in an unsatisfactory overall score.

Time began _____ **Time ended** _____

Steps	Possible Points	First Attempt	Second Attempt	Third Attempt
1. If warning is given that the patient feels faint, have the patient lower the head to the knees to increase blood supply to the brain. If this does not stop the episode, either have the patient lie down on the examination table or lower the patient to the floor. If the patient collapses to the floor when fainting, treat with caution due to possible head or neck injuries.	10			
2. Immediately notify the physician of the patient's condition and assess the patient for life-threatening emergencies such as respiratory or cardiac arrest. If the patient is breathing and has a pulse, monitor the patient's vital signs.	10			
3. Loosen any tight clothing and keep the patient warm, applying a blanket if needed.	20			
4. If there is no concern about a head or neck injury, elevate the patient's legs above the level of the heart.	10			
5. Continue to monitor vital signs and apply oxygen via nasal cannula if ordered by the physician.	10			

Steps	Possible Points	First Attempt	Second Attempt	Third Attempt
6. If vital signs are unstable or the patient does not respond quickly, activate emergency medical services.	10			
7. If the patient vomits, roll the patient on his or her side to avoid aspiration of vomitus into the lungs.	10			
8. Once the patient has completely recovered, assist the patient into a sitting position. *Do not* leave the patient unattended on the examination table.	10			
9. Document the incident including a description of the episode, patient symptoms, vital signs, length of time, and any complaints. If oxygen was administered, document the number of liters and length of administration.	10			

Documentation in the Medical Record

_____

_____

_____

_____

Comments:

Total Points Earned _____ Divided by _____ Total Possible Points = _____ % Score

Instructor's Signature _____

Procedure 24-6 Controlling Bleeding

Task: To stop hemorrhaging from an open wound.

Equipment and Supplies:
- Gloves, sterile if available
- Appropriate Personal Protective Equipment according to OSHA guidelines including:
  - Impermeable gown
  - Goggles
  - Impermeable mask
- Sterile dressings
- Bandaging material
- Biohazard waste container

Standards: Complete the procedure and all critical steps in _____ minutes with a minimum

score of _____ % within three attempts.

Scoring: Divide points earned by total possible points. Failure to perform a critical step that is indicated with an asterisk (*), will result in an unsatisfactory overall score.

Time began _____ **Time ended** _____

Steps	Possible Points	First Attempt	Second Attempt	Third Attempt
1. Wash hands and apply appropriate personal protective equipment.	10			
2. Assemble equipment and supplies.	10			
3. Apply several layers of sterile dressing material directly to the wound and exert pressure.	10			
4. Wrap the wound with bandage material. Add more dressing and bandaging material if bleeding continues.	10			
5. If bleeding persists and the wound is located on an extremity, elevate the extremity above the level of the heart. Notify the physician immediately if bleeding cannot be controlled.	10			
6. If bleeding still continues, apply pressure to the appropriate artery. If bleeding is in the arm, apply pressure to the brachial artery by squeezing the inner aspect of the upper mid-arm. If bleeding is in the leg apply pressure to the femoral artery on the affected side by pushing with the heel of the hand into the femoral crease at the groin. *If bleeding cannot be controlled, it may be necessary to activate the emergency medical system.*	10			

Steps	Possible Points	First Attempt	Second Attempt	Third Attempt
7. Once the bleeding is controlled and the patient is stabilized, dispose of contaminated materials into the biohazard waste container.	**10**	_____	_____	_____
8. Disinfect the area, remove gloves, and dispose into biohazard waste.	_____	_____	_____	_____
9. Wash hands.	**10**	_____	_____	_____
10. Document the incident including the details of the wound, when and how it occurred, patient symptoms, vital signs, physician treatment, and the patient's current condition	**10**	_____	_____	_____

Documentation in the Medical Record

_____

_____

_____

_____

Comments:

Total Points Earned _____ Divided by _____ Total Possible Points = _____ % Score

Instructor's Signature _____

Procedure 25-1 Preparing a Resumé

Task: To write an effective resume for use as a tool in gaining employment.

Equipment and Supplies:
• Scratch paper
• Pen or pencil
• Former job descriptions, if available
• List of addresses of former employers, schools, and names of supervisors
• Computer or word processor
• Quality stationary and envelopes

Standards: Complete the procedure and all critical steps in _____ minutes with a minimum

score of _____ % within three attempts.

Scoring: Divide points earned by total possible points. Failure to perform a critical step that is indicated with an asterisk (*), will result in an unsatisfactory overall score.

Time began _____ **Time ended** _____

Steps	Possible Points	First Attempt	Second Attempt	Third Attempt
1. Perform a self-evaluation by making notes about your strengths as a medical assistant. Consider job skills, self-management skills, and transferable skills.	10			
2. Explore formatting and decide on a professional resume appearance that best highlights your skills and experience. Use the templates available in word processing software or design your own.	10			
3. Place your name, address, and two telephone numbers where you can be contacted at the top of the resume.	10			
4. Write a job objective that specifies your employment goals.	10			
5. Provide details about your educational experience. List degrees and/or certifications obtained.	10			
6. Provide details about your work experience. Include all contact information and names of supervisors. Do not include salary expectations or reasons for leaving former jobs.	10			
7. Prepare a cover letter and a list of references. Send the references with the resume only when requested.	10			

Steps	Possible Points	First Attempt	Second Attempt	Third Attempt
8. Type the resume carefully and make certain that there are no errors on the document.	10			
9. Proofread the resume. Allow another person to read it as well and look for missed errors.*	5			
10. Print the resume on quality paper. Review the resume again for errors and to assure that it looks attractive on the printed page.	5			
11. Target each resume to a specific person or position. Do not send generic resumes to each prospective employer.	5			
12. Follow up on all resumes that are distributed with a phone call to arrange an interview.	5			

Documentation in the Medical Record

_____

_____

_____

_____

Comments:

Total Points Earned _____ Divided by _____ Total Possible Points = _____ % Score

Instructor's Signature _____

English-Spanish Terms for the Medical Assistant

academic degree A title conferred by a college, university, or professional school after completion of a program of study.
grado académico Título concedido por una, universidad o escuela profesional, tras completar un programa de estudios.

account A statement of transactions during a fiscal period and the resulting balance.
cuenta Estado de transacciones durante un periodo fiscal y el saldo resultante.

account balance The amount owed or on hand in an account.
saldo de la cuenta Suma que se debe o que está en una cuenta.

accounts receivable ledger A record of the income and payments due from creditors on an account.
libro mayor de cuentas por cobrar Registro de cargos y pagos asentados en una cuenta.

accreditation The process by which an organization is recognized for adhering to a group of standards that meet or exceed expectations of the accrediting agency.
acreditación Proceso por el cual se reconoce a una organización por su cumplimiento de ciertos estándares en un grado que cumple o sobrepasa las expectativas de la agencia que la acredita.

act The formal product of a legislative body; a decision or determination by a sovereign, a legislative council, or a court of justice.
ley Producto formal de un cuerpo legislativo; decisión o determinación por un soberano, un consejo legislativo o un tribunal de justicia.

adage A saying, often in metaphorical form, that embodies a common observation.
refrán Dicho, con frecuencia metafórico, que refleja una observación común.

advent A coming into being or use.
advenimiento Próximo a ser o a usarse.

advocate One who pleads the cause of another; one who defends or maintains a cause or proposal.
abogado Persona que defiende la causa de otro; aqel que defiende o apoya una causa o propuesta.

affable Being pleasant and at ease in talking to others; characterized by ease and friendliness.
afable Que es agradable y tiene un trato fácil con los demás; caracterizado por su trato fácil y amistoso.

agenda A list or outline of things to be considered or done.
agenda Lista o resumen de cosas a considerar o a hacer.

aggression A forceful action or procedure intended to dominate; hostile, injurious or destructive behavior, especially when caused by frustration.
agresión Acción o procedimiento **forzado**, con la intención de dominar; comportamiento hostil, injurioso o destructivo, en especial cuando es causado por frustración.

allegation A statement of what a party to a legal action undertakes to prove.
alegación Declaración por una de las partes implicadas en un proceso legal para apoyar lo que dicha parte intenta probar.

allied health fields Areas of healthcare delivery or related services in which professionals assist physicians with the diagnosis, treatment, and care of patients in many different specialty areas.
campos relacionados con la salud Áreas del cuidado de la salud y servicios relacionados en los cuales profesionales ayudan a los médicos en el diagnóstico, tratamiento y atención de los pacientes en muchas áreas diferentes.

allocating Apportioning for a specific purpose or to particular persons or things.
distribuir Asignar a un fin específico o a personas o cosas en particular.

allopathy A method of treating a disease by introducing a condition that is intended to cause a pathologic reaction, which will be antagonistic to the condition being treated.
alopatía Método de tratar una enfermedad provocando una afección con el fin de causar una reacción patológica, la cual será opuesta a la enfermedad que se está tratando.

allowed charge The maximum amount of money that many third-party payors will pay for a specific procedure or service. Often based on the UCR fee.
cargo permitido Cantidad máxima de dinero que muchos pagadores intermediarios pagan por una práctica o servicio específico; con frecuencia se basa en el cargo UCR.

alphabetic filing Any system that arranges names or topics according to the sequence of the letters in the alphabet.
archivo alfabético Cualquier sistema que ordena los nombres o temas siguiendo la secuencia de las letras del alfabeto.

alphanumeric Systems made up of combinations of letters and numbers.
alfanumérico Sistema constituido por combinaciones de letras y números.

ambiguous Capable of being understood in two or more possible senses or ways; unclear.
ambiguo Que puede entenderse de dos o más maneras; que no es claro.

ambulatory Able to walk about and not be bedridden.
ambulatorio Capaz de caminar y no tiene que estar postrado en la cama.

amenity Something conducive to comfort, convenience, or enjoyment.
amenidad Algo que proporciona confort, comodidad o placer.

ancillary diagnostic services Services that support patient diagnoses (e.g., laboratory or x-ray)
servicios de diagnóstico auxiliares Servicios que apoyan el diagnóstico del paciente (como laboratorio o rayos x).

ancillary Subordinate; auxiliary.
auxiliar Subordinado, complementario.

"and" In the context of ICD-9-CM, the word "and" should be interpreted as "and/or."
"y" En el contexto de ICD-9-CM, la palabra "y" debe interpretarse como "y/o".

animate Full of life; to give spirit and support to expressions.
animar Dar vida; dar ánimo y apoyo a las manifestaciones.

annotating To furnish with notes, which are usually critical or explanatory.
anotar Añadir notas, por lo general, críticas o explicatorias.

annotation A note added by way of comment or explanation.
anotación Nota añadida a modo de comentario o explicación.

appeal A legal proceeding by which a case is brought before a higher court for review of the decision of a lower court.
apelación Procedimiento legal por el cual un caso se lleva ante un tribunal superior para obtener una revisión de la decisión de un tribunal inferior.

appellate Having the power to review the judgment of another tribunal or body of jurisdiction, such as an appellate court.
de apelación Que tiene el poder de revisar el veredicto de otro tribunal o cuerpo jurídico, como una corte de apelación.

applications Software programs designed to perform specific tasks.
aplicaciones Programas informáticos diseñados para realizar tareas específicas.

appraisal To give an expert judgment of the value or merit of; judging as to quality.
evaluación Acción de emitir un juicio experto sobre el valor o mérito de algo; juzgar la calidad de algo; evaluar el rendimiento en el trabajo.

arbitration The hearing and determination of a cause in controversy by a person or persons either chosen by the parties involved or appointed under statutory authority.
arbitraje Vista y resolución de una causa en conflicto por una persona o personas elegida/s por las partes implicadas o designadas por la autoridad establecida por ley.

arbitrator A neutral person chosen to settle differences between two parties in a controversy.
árbitro Persona neutral seleccionada para poner fin a las diferencias entre dos partes involucradas en un conflicto.

archaic Of, relating to, or characteristic of an earlier or more primitive time.
arcaico Perteneciente o relativo a una época anterior o más primitiva; que tiene las características de dicha época.

archived To file or collect records or documents in or as if in an archive.
archivar Guardar o recoger informes o documentos en un archivo o de manera similar.

artificial intelligence The aspect of computer science that deals with computers taking on the attributes of humans. One such example is an expert system, which is capable of making decisions, like software that is designed to help a physician diagnose a patient, given a set of symptoms. Game-playing programming and programs designed to recognize human language are other examples of artificial intelligence.
inteligencia artificial Parte de la informática que se ocupa de la incorporación de atributos humanos a las computadoras. Un ejemplo de esto es un sistema práctico capaz de tomar decisiones, como los programas informáticos diseñados para ayudar a los médicos a diagnosticar a un paciente dado un conjunto de síntomas. Los programas de juegos y otros programas diseñados para reconocer el lenguaje humano son otros ejemplos.

ASCII American Standard Code for Information Interchange, a code representing English characters as numbers where each is given a number from 0 to 127.
ASCII Estándar Americano de Codificación para el Intercambio de Información; un código que representa carácteres ingleses como números, en el cual a cada uno se le asigna un número de 0 a 127.

assault An intentional, unlawful attempt to do bodily injury to another by force.
asalto Intento ilícito de causar daño físico a otro usando la fuerza.

assent To agree to something, especially after thoughtful consideration.
asentir Aceptar algo, especialmente cuando se hace tras una detenida reflexión.

asystole The absence of a heartbeat.
asistolia Ausencia de latidos del corazón.

authorization A term used by managed care for an approved referral.
autorización Término usado en el cuido administrado para referirse a la aprobación de la referencia de un paciente de un médico a otro profesional del cuidado o de la salud.

back-up Any type of storage of files to prevent their loss in the event of hard disk failure.
copia de seguridad Cualquier tipo de almacenamiento de archivos para evitar que se pierdan en caso de que ocurrra un fallo en el disco duro.

bailiff An officer of some U.S. courts, usually serving as a messenger or usher, who keeps order at the request of the judge.
alguacil Funcionario de algunos tribunales estadounidenses que suele servir como mensajero o ujier y que se ocupa de mantener el orden a petición del juez.

bank reconciliation The process of proving that a bank statement and checkbook balance are in agreement
reconciliación bancaria Proceso por el cual se prueba que un estado bancario y un saldo de una libreta de cheques concuerdan.

banners Banners, or banner ads, are advertisements often found on a webpage, which can be animated and attract the user's attention in hopes that he or she will click on the ad and be redirected to the advertiser's home page, and hence purchase from the site or gain information from the site.
viñetas Viñetas o anuncios de viñetas; anuncios, a **veces** animados, que se hallan, con frecuencia en las páginas web; su fin es atraer la atención del usuario con la esperanza de que éste haga clic en el anuncio, y así sea llevado a la página principal del anunciante para que compre algo en ese sitio o para que obtenga información sobre el mismo.

battery A willful and unlawful use of force or violence upon the person of another. An offensive touching or use of force on a person without that person's consent
golpiza Uso de la fuerza o violencia en contra de la persona de otro, de manera intencional e ilegítima. Tocar de manera ofensiva a una persona o usar la fuerza en contra de ella sin su consentimiento.

beneficence The act of doing or producing good, especially performing acts of charity or kindness.
beneficencia Acción de hacer o producir el bien, en especial llevando a cabo obras caritativas o bondadosas.

beneficiary The person receiving the benefits of an insurance policy. The "insured" person on a Medicare claim.
beneficiario Persona que recibe los beneficios de una póliza de seguro. La persona "asegurada" en una reclamación de Medicare.

benefits A service or payment provided under a health plan, employee plan, or some other agreement, including programs such as health insurance, pensions, retirement planning, and many other options that may be offered to employees of a company or organization.
beneficios Servicio o pago proporcionado bajo un plan de salud, un plan de empleados o algún otro acuerdo, incluyendo programas como seguros de salud, pensiones, planes de retiro y muchas otras opciones que pueden ser ofrecidas a los empleados de una compañía u organización.

benefits The amount payable by the insurance company for a monetary loss to an individual insured by that company, under each coverage.
beneficios Suma que ha de pagar la compañía aseguradora por una pérdida monetaria a un individuo asegurado por dicha compañía, bajo cada cobertura.

birthday rule When an individual is covered under two insurance policies, the insurance plan of the policyholder whose birthday comes first in the calendar year (month and day—not year) becomes primary.
regla del cumpleaños Cuando un individuo está cubierto bajo dos pólizas de seguro, el plan de seguro del titular de la póliza cuya fecha de cumpleaños esté antes en el año civil (mes y día, no año) se convierte en el plan primario.

blatant Completely obvious, conspicuous, or obtrusive, especially in a crass or offensive manner; brazen.
flagrante Completamente obvio, notorio o inoportuno, en especial de una manera torpe u ofensiva; desvergonzado.

bond A durable, formal paper used for documents.
obligación Papel duradero y formal usado para documentos.

burnout Exhaustion of physical or emotional strength or motivation, usually as a result of prolonged stress or frustration.
agotamiento Llegar al fin de la fortaleza o motivación física o emocional, por lo general como resultado un prolongado estado de estrés o frustración.

byte A unit of data that contains eight binary digits.
byte Unidad de información que contiene ocho dígitos binarios.

cache A special high-speed storage, which can be either part of the computer's main memory or a separate storage device. One function of cache is to store Web sites visited in the computer memory for faster recall the next time the Web site is requested.
caché Almacenamiento especial de alta velocidad que puede formar parte de la memoria principal de la computadora o puede ser un dispositivo de almacenamiento separado. Una función del caché es almacenar las páginas Web visitadas en la memoria de la computadora para llegar a ellas con mayor rapidez la próxima vez que desee ver la página.

caption A heading, title, or subtitle under which records are filed.
leyenda Encabezamiento, título o subtítulo bajo el cual se archivan los informes.

case management The process of assessing and planning patient care, including referral and follow-up to ensure continuity of care and quality management.
administración de casos Proceso de evaluación y planificación de la atención al paciente, incluyendo envío de pacientes a especialistas y seguimiento del caso para asegurar la continuidad del tratamiento y la calidad de la administración.

cash on delivery (COD) Method of payment used when an article or item is delivered, and payment is expected before it is released.
contra reembolso (COD) Método de pago usado cuando se entrega un artículo u objeto y el destinatario ha de pagar antes de recibirlo.

categorically Placed in a specific division of a system of classification.
categorizado Colocado en un lugar específico dentro de una división de un sistema de clasificación.

caustic A remark or phrase dripping with sarcasm.
cáustico Comentario o frase dicha con sarcasmo.

caustic A substance that burns or destroys tissue by chemical action.
cáustico Substancia que quema o destruye tejidos por acción química.

CD Burner A CD writer that is capable of writing data onto a blank CD, or copying data from a CD to another blank CD.
grabador de CD Dispositivo que puede escribir datos en un CD en blanco o copiar datos de un CD a otro CD en blanco.

certification Attested as being true, as represented, or as meeting a standard; to have been tested, usually by a third party, and awarded a certificate based on proven knowledge.
certificación Atestiguar que algo es verdadero en cuanto a lo que representa, o al cumplimiento de un estándar; que ha sido examinado, por lo general por una tercera parte, y que se le ha concedido un certificado basándose en el conocimiento del que ha dado prueba.

chain of command A series of executive positions in order of authority.
cadena de mando Serie de puestos ejecutivos en orden de autoridad.

channels A means of communication or expression; a way, course, or direction of thought.
canales Medios de comunicación o de expresión; vía, curso o dirección del pensamiento.

characteristic A distinguishing trait, quality, or property.
característica Rasgo, cualidad o propiedad distintiva.

chief complaint Reason for patient seeking medical care.
problema principal Razón por la cual un paciente solicita atención médica.

chiropractic A medical discipline in which a chiropractic physician focuses on the nervous system and manually and painlessly adjusts the vertebral column in order to affect the nervous system, resulting in healthier patients.
quiropráctica Disciplina médica en la que los médicos quiroprácticos se centran en el sistema nervioso y ajustan la columna vertebral manualmente y sin dolor, para lograr un efecto sobre el sistema nervioso, dando como resultado pacientes más sanos.

chronologic order Of, relating to, or arranged in or according to the order of time.
orden cronológico Perteneciente o relativo al orden en el tiempo; organizado según el orden en el tiempo.

circumvention To manage to avoid something, especially by ingenuity or stratagem.
circunvenir Lograr evitar algo usando ingeniosidad o estratagemas.

cite To quote by way of example, authority, or proof, or to mention formally in commendation or praise.
cita Que se nombra para servir de ejemplo, autoridad o prueba o para hacer una mención formal como recomendación o alabanza.

claims clearinghouse A centralized facility (sometimes called a third-party administrator or TPA) to whom insurance claims are transmitted, and who checks and redistributes claims electronically to various insurance carriers.
centro de reclamaciones Establecimiento centralizado (algunas veces conocido como administrador mediador o TPA) al cual se transmiten las reclamaciones de seguros y que se encarga de verificar y redistribuir las reclamaciones electrónicamente a varias compañías de seguros.

clarity The quality or state of being clear.
claridad Calidad o estado de claro.

clauses A group of words containing a subject and predicate and functioning as a member of a complex or compound sentence.
cláusulas Conjunto de palabras que incluye un sujeto y un predicado y que funciona como miembro de una oración compuesta.

clean claim An insurance claim form that has been completed correctly (with no errors or omissions) and can be processed and paid promptly.
reclamación limpia Formulario de reclamación de seguro que ha sido llenado correctamente (sin errores ni omisiones) y que puede procesarse y pagarse prontamente.

clearinghouses Networks of banks that exchange checks with each other.
sistema de compensación Redes bancarias que intercambian cheques entres sí.

clinical trials A research study that tests how well new medical treatments or other interventions work in the subjects, usually human beings.
ensayos clínicos Estudio de investigación que prueba cómo actúan los nuevos tratamientos médicos u otras intervenciones en los sujetos, normalmente en los seres humanos.

"code also" When more than one code is necessary to fully identify a given condition, "code also" of "use additional code" is used.
"código adicional" Cuando se necesita más de un código para identificar por completo una afección (enfermedad) determinado, se usa "código adicional" o "usar código adicional".

Code of Federal Regulations (CFR) The Code of Federal Regulations (CFR) is a coded delineation of the rules and regulations published in the Federal Register by the various departments and agencies of the federal government. The CFR is divided into 50 Titles, which represent broad subject areas, and further into chapters, which provide specific detail.
Código de Regulaciones Federales (CFR) El Código de Regulaciones Federales (CFR) es un resumen codificado de las normas y regulaciones publicadas en el Registro Federal por los diferentes departamentos y agencias del gobierno federal. El CFR se divide en 50 Títulos que representan amplias áreas temáticas, los cuales, a su vez, se subdividen en capítulos que proporcionan detalles específicos.

cohesive The state of sticking together tightly; exhibiting or producing the cohesion.
cohesivo El estado de estar estrechamente unidos; mostrar o producir cohesión.

comfort zone A place in the mind where an individual feels safe and confident.
zona de bienestar Un lugar en la mente en el que un individuo se siente seguro y confiado.

commensurate Corresponding in size, amount, extent, or degree; equal in measure.
equiparable Que es equivalente en tamaño, cantidad o grado; de igual medida.

commercial insurance Plans (sometimes called private insurance) that reimburse the insured (or his or her dependents) for monetary losses due to illness or injury according to a specific schedule as outlined in the insurance policy and on a fee-for-service basis. Individuals insured under these plans are normally not limited to any one physician and can usually see the health care provider of their choice.
seguro comercial Planes (a veces llamados seguros privados) que reembolsan al asegurado (o a sus dependendientes) por pérdidas monetarias debidas a enfermedad o lesión siguiendo una escala específica que se explica en la póliza de seguro y cobrando un cargo por cada servicio. Los individuos asegurados bajo estos planes, por lo general, no están limitados a un solo médico y suelen poder acudir al proveedor del cuidado de la salud que elijan.

comorbidities Preexisting conditions that will, because of their presence with a specific principal diagnosis, cause an increase in length of stay by at least 1 day in approximately 75 percent of cases.
patologías coexistentes Enfermedades preexistentes que, debido a su presencia junto al diagnóstico principal, causan un aumento en la duración de la estadía de al menos un día en aproximadamente 75 por ciento de los casos.

competence The quality or state of being competent; having adequate or requisite capabilities.
competencia Capacidad o aptitud de quien es competente en algo; tener las capacidades necesarias o cumplir con los requisitos necesarios para hacer algo.

competent Having adequate abilities or qualities; having the capacity to function or perform in a certain way.
competente Que tiene ciertas capacidades o cualidades; que tiene la capacidad de funcionar o actuar de un modo determinado.

complications Conditions that arise during the hospital stay that prolong the length of stay by at least 1 day in approximately 75 percent of the cases.
complicaciones Condiciones que surgen durante la permanencia en el hospital que prolongan el tiempo de la estadía en al menos un día en aproximadamente 75 por ciento de los casos.

computer A machine that is designed to accept, store, process, and give out information.
computadora (u ordenador) Máquina diseñada para aceptar, almacenar, procesar y emitir información.

concise Expressing much in brief form.
conciso Que expresa mucho en forma breve.

concurrently Occurring at the same time.
concurrente Que ocurre al mismo tiempo.

congruent Being in agreement, harmony, or correspondence; conforming to the circumstances or requirements of a situation.
congruente Que está en acuerdo, armonía o correspondencia; conforme a las circunstancias o requisitos de una situación.

connotation An implication; something suggested by a word or thing.
connotación Implicación; lo que sugiere una palabra o una cosa.

contamination To make impure or unclean; to make unfit for use by the introduction of unwholesome or undesirable elements.
contaminación Volver impuro o sucio; hacer que algo sea inadecuado para el uso por la introducción de elementos insalubres o indeseables.

continuation pages The second and following pages of a letter.
paginas de continuación En una carta, la segunda página y las siguientes.

continuing education credits (CEUs) Credits for courses, classes, or seminars related to an individual's profession, designed to promote education and to keep the professional up-to-date on current procedures and trends in his or her field; often required for licensing.
créditos de educación continua (CEU) Créditos por cursos, clases o seminarios relacionados con la profesión de un individuo y que tienen la finalidad de promocionar la educación y mantener al profesional al corriente de los procedimientos y tendencias actuales en su campo; con frecuencia son obligatorios para obtener una licencia.

continuity of care Care that continues smoothly from one provider to another so that the patient receives the most benefit and no interruption in care.
continuidad de la atención Atención que continúa sin interrupciones de un proveedor a otro, de manera que el paciente recibe los máximos beneficios sin que haya una interrupción de la atención sanitaria.

contributory negligence Statutes in some states that may prevent a party from recovering damages if he or she contributed in any way to the injury or condition.
negligencia concurrente Estatutos existentes en algunos estados que impiden que una parte sea recompensada por daños si esta parte ha contribuido en algún modo a provocar la lesión o enfermedad.

cookies A message that is sent to the Web browser from the Web server, which identifies users and can prepare custom Web pages for them, possibly displaying their name upon return to the site.
cookies Mensaje que se envía al navegador de la red desde el servidor, el cual identifica a los usuarios y puede preparar páginas web especiales para ellos, posiblemente, mostrando su nombre la próxima vez que visiten el sitio.

coordination of benefits The mechanism used in group health insurance to designate the order in which multiple carriers are to pay benefits to prevent duplicate payments.
coordinación de beneficios Mecanismo usado en seguros de enfermedad de grupo para designar el orden en el que varias compañías de seguros tienen que pagar los beneficios para evitar pagos dobles.

copayment A copayment (or coinsurance) is a policy provision frequently found in medical insurance, whereby the policyholder and the insurance company share the cost of *covered* losses in a specified ratio (i.e., 80/20–80 percent by the insurer and 20 percent by the insured).

co-pago Un co-pago (o co-seguro) es una provisión frecuente de la póliza en los seguros médicos, por la que el titular de la póliza y la compañía aseguradora comparten el costo de las pérdidas *cubiertas* en una proporción determinada (ej.: 80/20–80 por ciento por parte del asegurador y 20 por ciento por parte del asegurado).

counteroffer A return offer made by one who has rejected an offer or job.
contraoferta Oferta-respuesta hecha por quien ha rechazado una oferta o trabajo.

credentialing The act of extending professional or medical privileges to an individual; the process of verifying and evaluating that person's credentials.
concesión de credenciales Acción de conceder privilegios profesionales o médicos a un individuo; proceso de verificar y evaluar los credenciales de esa persona.

credibility The quality or power of inspiring belief.
credibilidad Calidad de creíble; facilidad para ser creído.

credit An entry on an account constituting an addition to a revenue, net worth, or liability account; the balance in a person's favor in an account.
crédito Dato que se entra en una cuenta y que constituye una adición a los ingresos, ganancia neta o cuenta de pasivo; saldo a favor de una persona en una cuenta.

critical thinking The constant practice of considering all aspects of a situation when deciding what to believe or what to do.
razonamiento crítico Práctica constante de considerar todos los aspectos de una situación al decidir qué creer o qué hacer.

cross-training Training in more than one area so that a multitude of duties may be performed by one person, or so that substitutions of personnel may be made when necessary or in emergencies.
entrenamiento cruzado Entrenamiento en más de un área, de modo que una persona pueda desempeñar varias labores o que se puedan realizar sustituciones de personal cuando sea necesario o en caso de emergencia.

cultivate To foster the growth of; to improve by labor, care, or study.
cultivar Promover el desarrollo; mejorar algo por medio de trabajo, cuidado o estudio.

cursor A symbol appearing on the monitor that shows where the next character to be typed will appear.
cursor Símbolo que aparece en el monitor y que muestra el lugar donde aparecerá el próximo carácter que se escriba.

curt Marked by rude or peremptory shortness.
cortante Caracterizado por una interrupción ruda o perentoria.

cyberspace A word used to describe the non-physical space of the online world of computer networks.
ciberespacio Palabra que se usa para describir el espacio no-físico del mundo en linea de las redes informáticas.

damages Loss or harm resulting from injury to person, property, or reputation; compensation in money imposed by law for losses or injuries.
daños Pérdidas o perjuicios que resultan de injuriar a una persona, atentar contra una propiedad o una reputación; compensación monetaria impuesta por ley en casos de pérdidas o injurias.

database A collection of related files that serves as a foundation for retrieving information.
base de datos Conjunto de archivos relacionados que sirven de base para la recuperación de información.

debit An entry on an account constituting an addition to an expense or asset balance, or a deduction from a revenue, net worth, or liability balance.
débito Dato que se entra en una cuenta y que constituye una adición a los gastos o a una cuenta de activo o una deducción de un ingreso, ganancia neta o cuenta de pasivo.

debit card A card similar to a credit card by which money may be withdrawn or the cost of purchases paid directly from the holder's bank account without the payment of interest.
tarjeta de débito Tarjeta similar a la de crédito pero con la cual se puede retirar dinero o pagar compras directamente de la cuenta bancaria del titular sin tener que pagar intereses.

decedent A legal term used to represent a deceased person.
difunto Término legal usado para referirse a una persona muerta.

decode To convert, as in a message, into intelligible form; to recognize and interpret.
decodificar Convertir la información, como en un mensaje, de modo que sea inteligible; reconocer e interpretar.

deductible A specific amount of money a patient must pay out-of-pocket, up front before the insurance carrier begins paying. Often this amount is in the range of from $100 to $1000. This deductible amount must be met on a yearly or per incident basis.
deducible Cantidad de dinero específica que un paciente debe pagar de su bolsillo antes de que la compañía de seguros comience a pagar. Con frecuencia esta suma está entre 100 y 1000 dólares. Esta cantidad deducible ha de satisfacerse anualmente o por caso.

default A failure to pay financial debts, especially a student loan.
incumplimiento Dejar de pagar deudas financieras, especialmente en un préstamo de estudiante.

defense mechanisms Psychological methods of dealing with stressful situations that are encountered in day-to-day living.
mecanismos de defensa Métodos psicológicos de hacer frente a situaciones tensas que surgen en la vida diaria.

deferment A postponement, especially of a student loan.
aplazamiento Postergación de un pago, especialmente en un préstamo de estudiante.

demeanor Behavior toward others; outward manner.
conducta Comportamiento hacia los demás; comportamiento que se exterioriza.

demographic The statistical characteristics of human populations (as in age or income), used especially to identify markets.
dato demográfico Característica estadística de la población humana (como edad o ingresos), que se usa sobre todo para identificar mercados.

detrimental Obviously harmful or damaging.
perjudicial Que es obvio que causa daño o perjuicio.

device driver The program or commands given to a device connected to a computer, which enable the device to function. For instance, a printer may come equipped with a software program that must be loaded onto the computer first, so that the printer will work.
controlador de dispositivo Programa que controla un dispositivo conectado a una computadora y que hace que dicho dispositivo pueda funcionar. Por ejemplo, una impresora puede estar equipada con un programa que primero ha de cargarse en la computadora para que ésta funcione.

diagnosis The determination of the nature of a disease, injury, or congenital defect.
diagnóstico Determinación del origen de una enfermedad, lesión o defecto congénito.

dictation The act or manner of uttering words to be transcribed.
dictado Acción de pronunciar palabras para que sean transcritas.

diction The choice of words, especially with regard to clearness, correctness, and effectiveness.
dicción Acción de elegir las palabras, especialmente para lograr claridad, corrección y eficacia en el discurso.

Digital Subscriber Lines (DSL) High speed, sophisticated modulation schemes that operate over existing copper telephone wiring systems; often referred to as "last-mile technologies" because DSL is used for connections from a telephone switching station to a home or office, and not between switching stations.
Línea de Abonado Digital (DSL) Sofisticado sistema de modulación de alta velocidad que opera en sistemas de cableado telefónicos de cobre ya existentes; con frecuencia se habla del DSL como "tecnología de las últimas millas" porque se utiliza para conexiones entre un centro de conmutación telefónica y un hogar u oficina, y no entre centros de conmutación.

Digital Versatile Disk (DVD) The DVD is an optical disk that holds approximately 28 times more information than a CD, and is most commonly used to hold full length movies.

Compared to a CD which holds approximately 600 megabytes, a DVD has the capacity to hold approximately 4.7 gigabytes.

Disco Digital Versátil (DVD) El DVD es un disco óptico con capacidad para almacenar unas 28 veces más información que un CD; su uso más común es para guardar películas de larga duración. Mientras que un CD puede almacenar unos 600 megabytes, un DVD tiene una capacidad aproximada de almacenamiento de 4.7 gigabytes.

dingy claim A claim that is put on hold because it lacks certain adjunction that allows it to be processed, often due to system changes.

reclamación oscura Reclamación en espera de ser procesada debido a que se necesita alguna información o elemento adicional, con frecuencia, debido a cambios en el sistema.

direct filing system A filing system in which materials can be located without consulting an intermediary source of reference.

sistema directo de archivo Sistema de archivo en el cual los materiales pueden ser localizados sin consultar una fuente de referencia intermedia.

dirty claim Claims that contain errors or omissions that cannot be processed or that must be processed by hand due to OCR scanner rejection.

reclamación sucia Reclamación con errores u omisiones que no puede procesarse o que debe procesarse manualmente debido a que el escáner OCR la rechaza.

disbursements Funds paid out.

desembolsos Dinero o fondos que se pagan.

discretion The quality of being discrete; having or showing good judgment or conduct, especially in speech.

discreción Calidad de discreto; tener sensatez o tacto al obrar, especialmente al hablar.

disk A magnetic surface that is capable of storing computer programs.

disco Superficie magnética capaz de almacenar programas de computadora.

disk drives Devices that load a program or data stored on a disk into the computer.

unidades de discos Dispositivos que cargan en la computadora un programa o datos almacenados en un disco.

disparaging Speaking slightingly about something or someone, with a negative or degrading tone.

menospreciar Hablar con desdén de algo o alguien, con un tono negativo o degradante.

disposition The tendency of something or someone to act in a certain manner under given circumstances.

disposición Tendencia de algo o alguien a actuar de un modo específico en determinadas circunstancias.

disruption A breaking down, or throwing into disorder.

disrupción Interrupción o creación de un estado de trastorno.

dissect To cut or separate tissue with a cutting instrument or scissors.

diseccionar Cortar o separar tejidos con tijeras u otro instrumento cortante.

dissection To separate into pieces and expose parts for scientific examination.

disección Separar en piezas y dejar las partes a la vista para realizar un estudio científico.

disseminate To disperse throughout.

diseminar Dispersar, esparcir.

disseminate To disburse; to spread around.

diseminado Suelto, esparcido.

docket A formal record of judicial proceedings; a list of legal causes to be tried.

orden del día Registro formal de procesos judiciales; lista de causas legales a juzgar.

domestic mail Mail that is sent within the boundaries of the United States and its territories.

correo nacional Correo que se envía dentro de los límites de Estados Unidos y sus territorios.

drawee Bank or facility on whom a check is drawn or written.

librado Banco o entidad contra la que se gira o emite un cheque.

due process A fundamental, constitutional guarantee that all legal proceedings will be fair, that one will be given notice of the proceedings and an opportunity to be heard before the government acts to take away life, liberty, or property; a constitutional guarantee that a law will not be unreasonable or arbitrary.

proceso debido Garantía fundamental constitucional de que todos los procesos legales serán justos, que las partes implicadas serán notificadas de los procedimientos y que se les dará la oportunidad de ser escuchados **rantes** que el gobierno les quite su vida, libertad o propiedad; garantía constitucional de que la ley no irá en contra de la razón ni será arbitraria.

duty Obligatory tasks, conduct, service, or functions that arise from one's position, as in life or in a group.

deber Tareas, conducta, servicio o funciones de carácter obligatorio que conlleva el ocupar un puesto, en la vida o como miembro de un grupo.

dyspnea Difficult or painful breathing.

disnea Respiración difícil o dolorosa.

e-banking Electronic banking via computer modem or over the Internet.

banca electrónica Operaciones bancarias a través del módem de una computadora o en Internet.

ecchymosis A hemorrhagic skin discoloration, commonly called bruising.

equimosis Descoloramient o hemorrágico de la piel comúnmente conocido como magulladura.

eCommerce A term used to describe the sale and purchase of goods and services over the Internet; doing business over the Internet; an abbreviation for "electric commerce."

comercio electrónico Expresión que se usa para describir la compra y venta de bienes y servicios a través de Internet; hacer negocios a través de Internet. Se conoce también con la abreviatura de comercio-e.

electronic claims Claims that are submitted to insurance processing facilities using a computerized medium such as direct data entry, direct wire, dial-in telephone digital fax, or personal computer download/upload.

reclamación electrónica Reclamaciones enviadas al lugar de procesamiento de la compañía aseguradora usando un sistema computarizado, tales como entrada de datos directa, cable directo, fax digital con marcado telefónico, o a través de una computadora personal.

e-mail Communications transmitted via computer using a modem.

correo electrónico Comunicaciones transmitidas a través de una computadora usando un módem.

emancipated minor A person under legal age who is self-supporting and living apart from parents or guardian.

menor emancipado Persona que no ha alcanzado la mayoría de edad legal y que se mantiene a sí misma y vive sin la custodia de padres o tutores.

embezzlement Stealing from an employer; appropriation without permission of goods, services, or funds for personal use.

desfalco Robo a un empleador; apropiación sin permiso de bienes, servicios o fondos para uso personal.

emetic A substance that causes vomiting.

emético Sustancia que causa vómito.

emisor Person who writes a check.

emisor Persona que emite un cheque.

empathy Sensitivity to the individual needs and reactions of patients.

empatía Sensibilidad ante las necesidades y reacciones individuales de los pacientes.

encode To convert from one system of communication to another; to convert a message into code.

codificar Convertir de un sistema de comunicación a otro; convertir un mensaje en un código.

encounter Any contact between a healthcare provider and a patient that results in treatment or evaluation of the patient's condition, not limited to in-person contact.

encuentro Cualquier contacto entre un proveedor de atención sanitaria y un paciente que resulta en un tratamiento o evaluación del estado del paciente; no se limita a un contacto personal.

encroachments To advance beyond the usual or proper limits.

intrusiones Ir más allá de los límites habituales o apropiados.

endorser Person who signs his or her name on the back of a check for the purpose of transferring title to another person.
endosante Persona que firma en la parte posterior de un cheque a fin de transferir la propiedad del mismo a otra persona.

enunciate To utter articulate sounds; the act of being very distinct in speech.
articular Pronunciar los sonidos de manera cuidada; hablar de una forma muy clara.

enunciation The utterane of articulate, clear sounds; the act of being very distinct in speech.
articulación Pronunciación cuidada, con sonidos claros.

established patients Patients who are returning to the office and who have previously seen the physician.
pacientes establecidos Pacientes que regresan al consultorio médico que ya han sido atendidos por el médico con anterioridad.

etiology Classifying a claim according to the cause of the disorder.
etiología Clasificación de una reclamación según la causa del trastorno.

euthanasia The act or practice of killing or permitting the death of hopelessly sick or injured individuals in a relatively painless way for reasons of mercy.
eutanasia Acción o práctica de matar o permitir la muerte de enfermos o heridos en estado terminal, de una forma relativamente sin dolor, por razones de piedad.

"excludes" Exclusion terms are always written in italics, and the word "Excludes" is enclosed in a box to draw particular attention to these instructions. Exclusion terms may apply to a chapter, a section, a category, or a subcategory. The applicable code number usually follows the exclusion term.
"excluye" Las expresiones de exclusión siempre se escriben en cursiva y la palabra "Excluye" se encierra en una casilla para llamar la atención acerca de estas instrucciones. Los términos de exclusión pueden ser aplicables a un capítulo, una sección, una categoría o una subcategoría. El número de código correspondiente por lo general sigue al término de exclusión.

expediency A situation requiring haste or caution; a means of achieving a particular end.
prontitud Situación que requiere actuar con prisa o precaución; un medio de alcanzar un fin específico.

expert witness A person who provides testimony to a court as an expert in a certain field or subject to verify facts presented by one or both sides in a lawsuit, often compensated and used to refute or disprove the claims of one party.
testigo perito Persona que da testimonio ante un tribunal como perito o experto en cierto campo o tema para verificar los hechos presentados por una o ambas partes en litigio, a menudo, cobrando una retribución económica, y cu yo testimonio suele usarse para refutar o impugnar las demandas de una de las partes.

external noise Noise outside the brain that interferes with the communication process.
ruido externo Ruido producido fuera del cerebro y que interfiere con el proceso de comunicación.

externalization To attribute an event or occurrence to causes outside the self.
exteriorización Acción de atribuir a un suceso o acontecimiento causas externas al mismo.

externship/internship A training program that is part of a course of study of an educational institution and is taken in the actual business setting in that field of study; these terms are often interchanged in reference to medical assisting.
prácticas internas/externas Programa de entrenamiento que es parte de un curso de estudio de una institución educativa y se sigue en un lugar real de trabajo en el campo de estudio; estos términos se intercambian cuando se refieren a los asistentes médicos.

fax Abbreviation for facsimile; a document sent using a fax machine.
fax Abreviatura de facsímile; documento que se envía usando una máquina de fax.

fee profile A compilation or average of physician fees over a given period of time.
perfil de cargo s Recopilación o porcentaje de cargos médicos en un periodo de tiempo dado.

fee schedule A compilation of preestablished fee allowances for given services or procedures.
escala de cargos Recopilación de asignaciones de cargos preestablecidos para servicios o procedimientos dados.

feedback The transmission of evaluative or corrective information to the original or controlling source about an action, event, or process.
reacciones y comentarios Envío de información de evaluación o corrección a la fuente original o a la que ejerce el control sobre una acción, suceso o proceso.

felony A major crime, such as murder, rape, or burglary; punishable by a more stringent sentence than that given for a misdemeanor.
crimen Delito mayor, como asesinato, violación o robo; se penaliza con una sentencia más severa que un delito menor o falta.

fermentation An enzymatically controlled transformation of an organic compound.
fermentación Transformación de un compuesto orgánico controlada por enzimas.

fervent Exhibiting or marked by great intensity of feeling.
ferviente Que posee sentimientos de gran intensidad o que da muestra de ellos.

fibrillation Rapid, random, ineffective contractions of the Herat.
fibrilación Contracciones cardiacas rápidas, aleatorias e inefectivas.

fidelity Faithfulness to something to which one is bound by pledge or duty.
fidelidad Fe en algo a lo que se está unido por juramento o deber.

fine A sum imposed as punishment for an offense; a forfeiture or penalty paid to an injured party or the government in a civil or criminal action.
multa Suma impuesta como penalización por un delito menor; suma que se paga a una parte a la que se ha perjudicado o dañado, o al gobierno, en un proceso civil o penal.

fiscal agent An organization or private plan under contract to the government to act as financial representatives in handling insurance claims from providers of health care; also referred to as fiscal intermediary.
agente fiscal Organización o plan privado bajo contrato con el gobierno para actuar como representantes financieros en la administración de reclamaciones de seguros por parte de proveedores de atención sanitaria; también se conoce como intermediario fiscal.

fiscal intermediary An organization that contracts with the government and other insuring entities to handle and mediate insurance claims from medical facilities.
intermediario fiscal Organización que establece un contrato con el gobierno y otras entidades aseguradoras para administrar reclamaciones de seguro provenientes de centros médicos y para mediar en ellas.

flagged Marked in some way so as to remind or remember that specific action needs to be taken.
señalado Marcado de alguna forma para recordar que se necesita que se tomen medidas al respeto.

flash Animation technology often used on the opening page of a Web site used to draw attention, excite, and impress the user.
flash Tecnología de imágenes animadas que se usa con frecuencia en la página inicial de un sitio web para llamar la atención del usuario, entusiasmarlo e impresionarlo.

flush Directly abutting or immediately adjacent, as set even with an edge of a type page or column; having no indention.
alineado Directamente contiguo o inmediatamente adyacente, ordenado de forma regular en relación con un borde de una página o columna; sin sangría o espacios en blanco.

font A design, as in typesetting, for a set of characters.
fuente tipográfica Diseño similar al de la composición para un conjunto de caracteres.

format To magnetically create tracks on a disk where information will be stored, usually done by the manufacturer of the disk.
formatear Crear pistas magnéticas en un disco destinado a almacenar información; por lo general, el fabricante del disco es quien se encarga de hacerlo.

gait Manner or style of walking.
andares Forma o estilo de caminar.

gamete A mature male or female germ cell, usually possessing a haploid chromosome set and capable of initiating formation of a new diploid individual.
gameto Célula germinal madura, tanto masculina como femenina, que por lo general tiene un conjunto cromosómico haploide y es capaz de iniciar la formación de un nuevo individuo diploide.

genome The genetic material of an organism.
genoma El material genético de un organismo.

genuineness Expressing sincerity and honest feeling.
autenticidad Expresión de sentimientos sincera y honrada.

gigabyte Approximately one billion bytes.
gigabyte Aproximadamente, mil millones de bytes.

girth A measure around a body or item.
contorno Medida alrededor de un cuerpo o artículo.

glean To gather information or material bit by bit; to pick over in search of relevant material.
recopilar Reunir información o material pedazo a pedazo; examinar en busca de material pertinente.

government plan An insurance or health care plan that is sponsored and/or subsidized by the state or federal government, such as Medicaid and Medicare.
plan del gobierno Seguro o plan de atención sanitaria patrocinado y subvencionado por el gobierno estatal o federal, como Medicaid y Medicare.

grammar The study of the classes of words, their inflections, and their functions and relations in the sentence; a study of what is to be preferred and what avoided in inflection and syntax.
gramática Estudio de las clases de palabras, sus desinencias y sus funciones y relaciones en la oración; estudio del uso que se prefiere y de lo que hay que evitar en cuanto a desinencias y sintaxis.

grief An unfortunate outcome; a deep distress caused by bereavement.
pesar Resultado desafortunado; profunda aflicción causada por la pérdida de un ser querido.

group policy Insurance written under a policy that covers a number of people under a single master contract issued to their employer or to an association with which they are affiliated.
póliza de grupo Seguro contratado bajo una póliza que cubre a varias personas bajo un único contrato maestro establecido con su empleador o con una asociación a la que estén afiliados.

guarantor A person who makes or gives a guarantee of payment for a bill.
garante Persona que paga una factura o que garantiza su pago.

guardian ad litem Legal representative for a minor.
tutor ad litem Representante legal de un menor.

hard copy The readable paper copy or printout of information.
copia impresa Copia impresa en papel o impresión de la información.

harmonious Marked by accord in sentiment or action; having the parts agreeably related.
armonioso Caracterizado por una armonía en los sentimientos o acciones; partes de un todo relacionadas de forma agradable.

health insurance Protection in return for periodic premiums, which provides reimbursement of monetary losses due to illness or injury. Included under this heading are various types of insurance such as accident insurance, disability income insurance, medical expense insurance, and accidental death and dismemberment insurance. Also known as accident and health insurance or disability income insurance.
seguro de enfermedad Cobertura a cambio del pago de primas periódicas, la cual proporciona el reembolso de las pérdidas monetarias debidas a enfermedad o lesión. Bajo este nombre se incluyen varios tipos de seguros como seguro de accidente, seguro de incapacidad, seguro de gastos médicos y seguro en caso de muerte y pérdida de extremidades. También se conoce como seguro de accidente y enfermedad o seguro de incapacidad.

HMO An organization that provides a wide range of comprehensive health care services for a specified group at a fixed periodic payment. HMOs can be sponsored by the government, medical schools, hospitals, employers, labor unions, consumer groups, insurance companies, and hospital-medical plans.
HMO Organización que proporciona una amplia gama de servicios completos de atención sanitaria

para un grupo específico por un pago periódico fijado. Las HMO puedes estar patrocinadas por el gobierno, facultades de medicina, hospitales, patronos, sindicatos laborales, grupos de consumidores, compañías aseguradoras y planes médico-hospitalarios.

holder Person presenting a check for payment.
portador Persona que presenta un cheque para cobrarlo.

holistic Related to or concerned with all of the systems of the body, rather than breaking it down into parts.
holístico Relacionado con todos los sistemas corporales y no dividido en partes.

HTML Abbreviation for hypertext markup language, which is the language used to create documents for use on the Internet.
HTML Abreviatura de lenguaje de marcas de hipertexto, que es el lenguaje que se emplea para crear documentos destinados a usarse en Internet.

HTTP Abbreviation for hypertext transfer protocol, which defines how messages are defined and transmitted over the Internet; when a URL is entered into the computer, an HTTP command tells the Web server to retrieve the requested Web page.
HTTP Abreviatura de protocolo de transporte de hipertexto, que define cómo se interpretan y transmiten los mensajes en Internet; cuando un URL entra en la computadora, una orden de HTTP manda la señal al servidor web para que busque la página web que se solicita.

Hub A common connection point for devices in a network containing multiple ports, often used to connect segments of a LAN.
Nodo Punto de conexión común para dispositivos en una red de conexiones de varios puertos; suele usar se para conectar segmentos de una LAN (red de área local).

icon A picture, often on the desktop of a computer, which represents a program or object. By clicking on the icon, the user is directed to the program.
icono Dibujo, con frecuencia colocado en el escritorio de la computadora, que representa un programa o un objeto. Al hacer clic sobre el icono, el usuario es llevado a dicho programa.

idealism The practice of forming ideas or living under the influence of ideas.
idealismo Práctica de formarse ideas o vivir bajo la influencia de ideas.

immigrant A person who comes to a country to take up permanent residence.
inmigrante Persona que va a un país para vivir allí de forma permanente.

impenetrable Incapable of being penetrated or pierced; not capable of being damaged or harmed.
impenetrable Que no puede ser penetrado o traspasado; que no puede ser dañado o perjudicado.

implied consent Presumed consent, such as when a patient offers an arm for a phlebotomy procedure.
consentimiento tácito Consentimiento que se supone que ha sido dado, como cuando un paciente presenta el brazo para que se le extraiga sangre.

incentive Something that incites or spurs to action; a reward or reason for performing a task.
incentivo Algo que incita o impulsa a actuar; recompensa o razón para llevar a cabo una tarea.

"includes" The appearance of this term under a subdivision such as a category (three-digit code) or two-digit procedure code, indicates that the code and title include these terms. Other terms also classified to that particular code and title are listed in the Alphabetic Indexes.
"incluye" La presencia de esta expresión, cuando aparece bajo una subdivisión, como una categoría (código de tres dígitos) o como un código de procedimiento de dos dígitos, indica que el código y el título incluyen estos términos. En los Índices alfabéticos se enumeran otros términos también clasificados para este código específico.

indemnity plan Traditional health insurance plan that pays for all or a share of the cost of covered services, regardless of which doctor, hospital, or other licensed health care provider is used. Policyholders of indemnity plans and their dependents choose when and where to get health care services.
plan de indemnización Plan de seguro de enfermedad tradicional que paga todo o parte del costo de los servicios que cubre, sin importar a qué médico, hospital u otro proveedor de atención sanitaria licenciado se acuda. Los titulares de pólizas de planes de indemnización y las personas

que dependen de estos titulares escogen cuándo y dónde recibir atención médica.

indicators An important point or group of statistical values that, when evaluated, indicate the quality of care provided in a healthcare institution.
indicadores Importante punto o grupo de valores estadísticos que al ser evaluados indican la calidad del servicio que se proporciona en una institución de atención sanitaria.

indicted To charge with a crime by the finding or presentment of a jury with due process of law.
acusado Que se le imputa con un cargo criminal por conclusión o acusación de un jurado con el proceso legal debido.

indigent Totally lacking in something of need.
indigente Que carece totalmente de algo necesario.

indirect filing system A filing system in which an intermediary source of reference, such as a card file, must be consulted to locate specific files.
sistema indirecto de archivo Sistema de archivo en el cual debe consultarse una fuente de referencia intermedia, como un fichero, para localizar documentos específicos.

individual policy An insurance policy designed specifically for the use of one person (and his or her dependents) not associated with the amenities of a group policy, namely higher premiums. Often referred to as "personal insurance."
póliza individual Póliza de seguros destinada específicamente a ser usada por una persona (y quienes dependan de ella) y que no conlleva los beneficios de una póliza de grupo y tiene primas más altas. Con frecuencia se le llama "seguro personal".

inflection A change in pitch or loudness of the voice.
inflexión Cambio en el tono o volumen de la voz.

informed consent A consent in which there is understanding of what treatment is to be undertaken and of the risks involved, why it should be done, and alternative methods of treatment available (including no treatment) and their attendant risks.
consentimiento informado Consentimiento que implica la comprensión del tratamiento al que se va a ser sometido y de los riesgos que conlleva, del porqué de dicho tratamiento, así como la

comprensión de los tratamientos alternativos disponibles (incluyendo la ausencia de tratamiento) y los riesgos que conllevan.

infraction Breaking the law; a minor offense of the rules.
infracción Incumplimiento de la ley; delito menor contra las normas establecidas.

initiative The causing or facilitating of the beginning of; the initiation of something into happening.
iniciativa El causar o facilitar el comienzo de algo; el hacer que algo comience a ocurrir.

innate Existing in, belonging to, or determined by factors present in an individual since birth.
innato Que existe en un individuo, que le pertenece o que está determinado por factores existentes en ese individuo desde el momento de su nacimiento.

input Information entered into and used by the computer.
entrada Información introducida en una computadora y que la computadora utiliza.

instigate To goad or urge forward; provoke.
instigar Incitar, exhortar, provocar.

insubordination Disobedience to authority.
insubordinación Desobediencia a la autoridad.

insured A person or organization who is covered by an insurance policy, along with any other parties for whom protection is provided under the policy terms.
asegurado Persona u organización que está cubierta por una póliza de seguro junto con cualquier otro a quien se proporcione cobertura bajo los términos de la póliza.

intangible Incapable of being perceived, especially by touch; incapable of being precisely identified or realized by the mind.
intangible Que no se puede percibir, especialmente que no se puede tocar; que no puede ser identificado con precisión ni ser comprendido por la mente.

integral Essential; being an indispensable part of a whole.
integral Esencial; parte indispensable de un todo.

interaction A two-way communication; mutual or reciprocal action or influence
interacción Comunicación bidireccional; acción o influencia recíproca o mutua.

intercom A two-way communication system with a microphone and loudspeaker at each station for localized use.
intercomunicador Sistema de comunicación bidireccional con un micrófono y un altavoz en cada estación para uso local.

intermittent Coming and going at intervals; not continuous
intermitente Que va y viene a intervalos; de forma no continua.

internal noise Noise inside the brain that interferes with the communication process.
ruido interno Ruido en el interior del cerebro que interfiere con el proceso de comunicación.

International Classification of Diseases, Ninth Revision, Clinical Modification (ICD-9-CM) System for classifying disease to facilitate collection of uniform and comparable health information for statistical purposes, and for indexing medical records for data storage and retrieval.
Clasificación Internacional de Enfermedades, Novena Revisión, Modificación clínica (ICD-9-CM) Sistema de clasificación de enfermedades para facilitar la recopilación de información médica uniforme, tanto para fines estadísticos como para indexar informes médicos a fin de almacenar y recuperar datos.

International Classification of Diseases, Tenth Revision (ICD-10) System containing the greatest number of changes in ICD's history. To allow more specific reporting of disease and newly recognized conditions, the ICD-10 contains approximately 5,500 more codes than ICD-9.
Clasificación Internacional de Enfermedades, Décima Revisión (ICD-10) Sistema que contiene el mayor número de cambios en la historia de la ICD. Para permitir elaborar informes más precisos de las enfermedades y de los estados patológicos que se conocen sólo recientemente, la ICD-10 incluye aproximadamente 5,500 códigos más que la ICD-9.

international mail Mail that is sent outside the boundaries of the United States and its territories.
correo internacional Correo que se envía fuera de los límites de Estados Unidos y sus territorios.

interval Space of time between events.
intervalo Espacio de tiempo entre dos sucesos.

intolerable Not tolerable or bearable.
intolerable Que no se puede tolerar o soportar.

intrinsic Belonging to the essential nature or constitution of a thing; indwelling, inward.
intrínseco Que pertenece a la naturaleza o constitución básica de una cosa; inherente, interno.

introspection An inward, reflective examination of one's own thoughts and feelings.
introspección Examen de nuestros propios pensamientos y sentimientos.

invariably Consistently; without changing or being capable of change.
invariablemente De forma constante; que no cambia ni puede cambiar.

invasive Involving entry into the living body, as by incision or insertion of an instrument.
invasivo Que entra en un organismo vivo, como por incisión o inserción de un instrumento.

jargon The technical terminology or characteristic idiom of a particular group or special activity.
jerga Terminología técnica o lenguaje característico de un grupo específico o una actividad especial.

java An object-oriented high-level programming language commonly used and well-suited for the Internet.
java Lenguaje de programación de alto nivel y orientado a objetos que es usado ampliamente y es muy adecuado para Internet.

judicial Of or relating to a judgment, the function of judging, the administration of justice, or the judiciary.
judicial Perteneciente o relativo al juicio, los procesos jurídicos, la administración de justicia o a la judicatura.

jurisdiction A power constitutionally conferred upon a judge or magistrate, to decide cases according to law and to carry sentence into execution. Jurisdiction is original when it is conferred on the court in the first instance (original jurisdiction); it is appellate when an appeal is given from the judgment of another court (apellate jurisdiction).
jurisdicción Poder constitucional otorgado a un juez o magistrado para resolver casos de acuerdo con la ley y hacer que se cumplan las sentencias. Es jurisdicción original cuando se otorga en un tribunal de primera instancia; es jurisdicción en apelación cuando existe una apelación al juicio de otro tribunal.

jurisprudence The science or philosophy of law; a system or body of law, or the course of court decisions.
jurisprudencia Ciencia o filosofía que trata sobre la ley; sistema o cuerpo legal; línea de decisiones de los tribunales.

language barrier Any type of interference that inhibits the communication process and is related to the difference in languages spoken by the people attempting to communicate.
barrera del idioma Cualquier tipo de interferencia que inhibe el proceso de comunicación y que está relacionado con la diferencia en los idiomas que hablan las personas que intentan comunicarse.

law A binding custom or practice of a community; a rule of conduct or action prescribed or formally recognized as binding or enforceable by a controlling authority.
ley Costumbre o práctica obligatoria de una comunidad; norma de comportamiento o proceder prescrita o reconocida formalmente como norma obligatoria o que se puede hacer cumplir por una autoridad encargada.

learning style The way that an individual perceives and processes information in order to learn new material.
estilo de aprendizaje Forma en la que un individuo percibe y procesa la información para aprender cosas nuevas.

liable Obligated according to law or equity; responsible for an act or circumstance.
responsable Que tiene alguna obligación según la ley o el derecho lato; responsable de un acto o circunstancia.

libel A written defamatory statement or representation that conveys an unjustly unfavorable impression.
libelo Escrito difamatorio que produce una impresión desfavorable injusta.

litigious Prone to engage in lawsuits.
litigioso Propenso a iniciar pleitos y litigios.

maker (of a check) Any individual, corporation, or legal party who signs a check or any type of negotiable instrument.
signatario (de un cheque) Cualquier individuo, corporación o parte legal que firma un cheque o cualquier tipo de instrumento negociable.

managed care An umbrella term for all health care plans that provide health care in return for preset monthly payments and offer coordinated care through a defined network of primary care physicians and hospitals.
atención administrada Término que engloba todos los planes de atención sanitaria que proporcionan atención médica a cambio de pagos mensuales preestablecidos y atención coordinada a través de una red definida de médicos de cabecera y hospitales.

mandated Required by an authority or law.
obligatorio Que lo exige una autoridad o la ley.

mandatory Containing or constituting a command.
obligatorio Que contiene una orden o que es una orden en sí mismo.

manifestation Something that is easily understood or recognized by the mind.
manifestación Algo que puede ser comprendido o reconocido por la mente con facilidad.

matrix Something in which a thing originates, develops, takes shape, or is contained; a base upon which to build.
matriz Algo donde las cosas se originan, desarrollan, toman forma o están contenidas; base sobre la cual construir.

m-banking Banking through the use of wireless devices, such as cellular phones and wireless internet services.
banca-m Operaciones bancarias a través de dispositivos inalámbricos, como teléfonos celulares y servicios de comunicaciones inalámbricas.

media The term applied to agencies of mass communication, such as newspapers, magazines, and telecommunications.
medios de comunicación Término que se aplica a las agencias de noticias o de comunicación de masas, como periódicos, revistas y telecomunicaciones.

mediastinum The space in the center of the chest, under the sternum.
mediastino Espacio en el centro del pecho, bajo el esternón.

medical savings account A tax-deferred bank or savings account combined with a low-premium/high-deductible insurance policy, designed for individuals or families who choose to fund their own health care expenses and medical insurance.

cuenta de ahorros para gastos médicos Cuenta bancaria o de ahorros de impuestos diferidos combinada con una póliza de seguro con primas bajas y deducibles altos destinada a individuos o familias que eligen financiar ellos mismos sus gastos de atención sanitaria y su seguro médico.

medically indigent An individual who can afford to pay for his or her normal daily living expenses but cannot afford adequate health care.

médicamente indigente Individuo que puede pagar sus gastos normales de la vida cotidiana pero que no puede abordar el pago de un servicio de atención sanitaria adecuado.

medically necessary Criteria used by third-party payors to decide whether a patient's symptoms and diagnosis justify specific medical services or procedures; also known as medical necessity.

médicamente necesario Criterio usado por pagadores intermediarios para decidir si los síntomas y el diagnóstico de un paciente justifican el uso de procedimientos o servicios médicos específicos; también se conoce como necesidad médica.

medigap A term sometimes applied to private insurance products that supplement Medicare insurance benefits.

medigap Término que se aplica algunas veces a seguros privados que complementan los beneficios del seguro Medicare.

megabyte Approximately one million bytes.

megabyte Aproximadamente, un millón de bytes.

megahertz A measuring unit for microprocessors, abbreviated MHz. A megahertz is a million cycles of electromagnetic current alternation per second and is used as a unit of measure for the clock speed of computer microprocessors. The hertz is a unit of measure named after Heinrich Hertz, a German physicist.

megahercio Unidad de medida para microprocesadores, abreviada MHz. Un megahercio es un millón de ciclos de alternancia de corriente electromagnética por segundo y se usa como unidad de medida para la velocidad de los microprocesadores de computadoras. El hercio recibe su nombre de Heinrich Hertz, un físico alemán.

mentor A trusted counselor or guide.

mentor Consejero o guía de confianza.

meticulous Marked by extreme or excessive care in the consideration or treatment of details.

meticuloso Caracterizado por una atención exagerada o excesiva a los detalles.

microfilm A film bearing a photographic record of printed or other graphic matter on a reduced scale.

microfilm Película que contiene una fotografía de un documento impreso u otro elemento gráfico a escala reducida.

MIDI The abbreviation for musical instrument digital interface. A MIDI interface allows computers to record and manipulate sound.

MIDI Abreviatura para interfaz digital para instrumentos musicales. Una interfaz MIDI permite a las computadoras grabar y manipular sonido.

misdemeanor A minor crime, as opposed to a felony, punishable by fine or imprisonment in a city or county jail rather than in a penitentiary.

falta Delito menor, por oposición a delito mayor, se penaliza con multa o prisión en una cárcel de una ciudad o condado más bien que con prisión en una penitenciaría.

mock To imitate or practice.

simular Imitar o practicar.

modem The acronym for modulator demodulator; a device that allows information to be transmitted over phone lines, at speeds measured in bits per second (bps).

módem Abreviatura para modulador desmodulador, un dispositivo que permite transmitir información a través de las líneas telefónicas a velocidades que se miden en bits por segundos (bps).

morale The mental and emotional condition (such as enthusiasm, confidence, or loyalty) of an individual or group with regard to the function or tasks at hand.

moral Estado mental y emocional (como entusiasmo, lealtad o confianza) de un individuo o grupo en cuanto al puesto que desempeña o el trabajo que realiza.

motivation The process of inciting a person to some action or behavior.

motivación Proceso de incitar a una persona a hacer algo o a comportarse de una forma determinada.

multimedia The presentation of graphics, animation, video, sound, and text on a computer in an integrated way, or all at once. CD-ROMs are the most effective multimedia devices.
multimedia Presentación de gráficos, imágenes animadas, video, sonido y texto en una computadora de forma integrada o simultánea. Los CD ROM son los dispositivos de multimedia más eficaces.

multi-tasking Performing multiple tasks at one time.
multitarea Realización de varias tareas diferentes al mismo tiempo.

municipal court A court that sits in some cities and larger towns and that usually has civil and criminal jurisdiction over cases arising within the municipality.
Municipal corte Se aplica al juzgado con sede en algunas ciudades y pueblos grandes y que suele tener jurisdicción civil y penal sobre casos que surgen dentro de la municipalidad.

mysticism The experience of seeming to have direct communication with God or ultimate reality.
misticismo Experiencia de parecer tener comunicación directa con Dios o una realidad superior.

naturopathy An alternative to conventional medicine in which holistic methods are used, as well as herbs and natural supplements, with the belief that the body will heal itself. Naturopathic physicians can currently be licensed in twelve states.
naturopatía Alternativa a la medicina convencional en la que se usan métodos holísticos, así como hierbas y suplementos naturales, con la creencia de que el cuerpo sanará por sí mismo. En la actualidad, los médicos naturópatas pueden obtener la licencia en doce estados.

negligence Failure to exercise the care that a prudent person usually exercises; implied inattention to one's duty or business; implied want of due or necessary diligence or care.
negligencia Falta de cuidado en algo que se hace; falta implícita de atención en el deber o trabajo; deseo implícito de una diligencia o cuidado necesario o merecido.

negotiable Legally transferable to another party.
negociable Que se puede transferir legalmente a otra parte.

networking The exchange of information or services among individuals, groups, or institutions; meeting and getting to know individuals in the same or similar career fields, and sharing information about available opportunities.
interconexión Intercambio de información o servicios entre individuos, grupos o instituciones; conocer a individuos del mismo campo profesional o de campos similares y compartir información acerca de oportunidades de empleo.

nonmaleficence Refraining from the act of harming or committing evil.
ausencia de maleficencia No hacer el mal.

no-show A person who fails to keep an appointment without giving advance notice.
no-acudió Persona que no acude a una cita médica sin dar previo aviso.

nosocomial infection Infection acquired during hospitalization or in a healthcare setting. It is often due to *E. coli*, hepatitis viruses, *pseudomonas*, and staphylocci microorganisms.
infección nosocomial Infección adquirida en un establecimiento de atención sanitaria o durante una hospitalización. Con frecuencia se debe a *E. coli*, virus de hepatitis, *pseudomonas* y estafilococos.

nosocomial Pertaining to or originating in the hospital, said of an infection not present or incubating prior to admission to the hospital.
nosocomial Perteneciente o relativo al hospital, incubado en el hospital, dícese de la infección que no estaba presente ni en estado de incubación antes de ser ingresado al hospital.

"note" Notes are found in both the Alphabetic Index and the Tabular List as instructions or guides in classification assignments, defining category content or the use of subdivision codes.
"nota" Las notas se encuentran tanto en los Índices alfabéticos como en las instrucciones o guías en las Asignaciones de clasificación, para definir el contenido de la categoría o el uso de los códigos de subdivisión.

objective information Information that is gathered by watching or observating a patient.
información objetiva Información que se recoge vigilando u observando a un paciente.

obliteration Making something indecipherable or imperceptible by obscuring or wearing away.
obliterar Hacer algo indescifrable o imperceptible oscureciéndolo o desgastándolo.

"omit code" This term is used primarily in Volume 3 when the procedure is the method of approach for an operation.
"omitir código" Esta expresión se usa sobre todo en el tomo 3 cuando el procedimiento es el método de acercamiento a una operación.

opinion A formal expression of judgment or advice by an expert; the formal expression of the legal reasons and principles upon with a legal decision is based.
opinión Expresión formal de un juicio o consejo dado por un experto; expresión formal de las razones y principios legales sobre los que se basa una decisión legal.

optical character recognition (OCR) The electronic scanning of printed items as images, then using special software to recognize these images (or characters) as ASCII text.
reconocimiento óptico de caracteres (OCR) Proceso de escanear electrónicamente documentos impresos como si fueran imágenes y después, usando un programa de computadora especial, reconocer esas imágenes (o caracteres) como texto ASCII.

ordinance An authoritative decree or direction; a law set forth by a governmental authority, specifically a municipal regulation.
ordenanza Decreto u orden de la autoridad; ley definida por una autoridad gubernamental, específicamente, una regulación municipal.

osteopathy A medical discipline based primarily on the manual diagnosis and holistic treatment of impaired function resulting from loss of movement in all kinds of tissues.
osteopatía Disciplina médica que se basa primordialmente en el diagnóstico manual y el tratamiento holístico de funciones deterioradas como resultado de la pérdida de movilidad en todo tipo de tejidos.

OUTfolder A folder used to provide space for the temporary filing of materials.
Carpeta OUT Carpeta que se usa para proporcionar espacio para archivar materiales de forma temporal.

OUTguide A heavy guide that is used to replace a folder that has been temporarily moved from the filing space.
Guía OUT Guía grande que se usa para reemplazar una carpeta que ha sido retirada temporalmente del archivo.

output Information that is processed by the computer and transmitted to a monitor, printer, or other device.
Salida Información procesada por la computadora y enviada a un monitor, impresora u otro dispositivo.

pandemic Affecting the majority of the people in a country or a number of countries.
pandémico Que afecta a la mayoría de la población de un país o de varios países.

paper claims Hard copies of insurance claims that have been completed and sent by surface mail.
reclamaciones de papel Copias impresas de reclamaciones de seguros que han sido completadas y enviadas por correo ordinario.

paraphrased Pertaining to a text, passage, or work that has been restated to give the meaning in another form.
parafraseado Perteneciente o relativo a un texto, selección u obra que ha sido expresado nuevamente para dar su significado de otra forma.

paraphrasing Expressing an idea in different wording in an effort to enhance communication and clarify meaning.
parafrasear Expresar una idea con palabras diferentes para mejorar la comunicación y hacer más claro su significado.

participating provider A physician or other health care provider who enters into a contract with a specific insurance company or program, and by doing so, agrees to abide by certain rules and regulations set forth by that particular third-party payor.
proveedor participante Médico u otro proveedor de atención sanitaria que establece un contrato con una compañía o programa de seguro específico, y al hacerlo acepta respetar ciertas normas y regulaciones establecidas por ese pagador intermediario.

payables The balance due to a creditor on an account.
pendiente de pago Saldo que se le debe al acreedor en una cuenta.

payee The person named on a draft or check as the recipient of the amount shown.
beneficiario Persona que se nombra en una letra de cambio o en un cheque como receptor de la cantidad indicada.

payer The person who writes a check to be cashed by the payee.
pagador Persona que emite el cheque a ser cambiado por el beneficiario.

peer review organization A group of medical reviewers who are contracted by HCFA to ensure quality control and the medical necessity of services provided by a facility.
organizacione de revisión colegial Grupo de revisores médicos contrata dos por HCFA para garantizar el control de calidad y la necesidad médica de los servicios ofrecidos por un establecimiento.

pegboard system A method of tracking patient accounts that allows the figures to be proven accurate by using mathematical formulas; also called the "write-it-once" system.
sistema de tablero perforado Método de controlar las cuentas de los pacientes que permite la demostración de la exactitud de las cifras por medio de fórmulas matemáticas; también conocido como sistema "escríbelo una vez."

perceiving The process of an individual looking at information and seeing it as real.
percibir Proceso en el cual un individuo mira la información y la ve como real.

perception A quick, acute, and intuitive cognition; capacity for comprehension; an awareness of the elements of the environment.
percepción Conocimiento rápido, agudo e intuitivo; capacidad de comprensión; conocimiento de los elementos del medio ambiente.

perjured testimony Testimony involving the voluntary violation of an oath or vow, either by swearing to what is untrue or by failing to do what has been promised under oath; false testimony.
perjuro Testimonio que comprende la violación voluntaria de un juramento o promesa, ya sea jurando algo que es falso o no cumpliendo lo que se ha prometido bajo juramento; falso testimonio.

perks Extra advantages or benefits from working in a specific job that may or may not be commonplace in that particular profession.
beneficios adicionales Ventajas o beneficios adicionales del trabajar en un puesto de trabajo específico que pueden ser o no comunes a esa profesión en particular.

persona An individual's social facade or front that reflects the role the individual is playing in life; the personality that a person projects in public.
persona Lo que vemos de un individuo, la imagen social que refleja el papel que dicho individuo tiene en la sociedad; la personalidad que una persona proyecta en público.

pertinent Having a clear, decisive relevance to the matter at hand.
pertinente Que tiene una importancia clara y decisiva en el asunto que se está tratando.

philanthropist An individual who makes an active effort to promote human welfare.
filántropo Individuo que se ocupa activamente de promover el bienestar humano.

philosopher A person who seeks wisdom or enlightenment; an expounder of a theory in a certain area of experience.
filósofo Persona que busca la sabiduría o el esclarecimiento; persona que expone una teoría en cierta área de experiencia.

phonetic Describing an alteration of ordinary spelling that better represents the spoken language, that employs only characters of the regular alphabet, and that is used in a context of conventional spelling.
escritura fonética Alteración de la escritura normal que representa mejor el lenguaje hablado, emplea sólo caracteres del alfabeto normal y se usa en un contexto de escritura convencional.

photophobia Abnormal visual sensitivity to light.
fotofobia Sensibilidad visual anómala a la luz.

physiological noise Physiological interference with the communication process.
ruido fisiológico Interferencia fisiológica con el proceso de comunicación.

pitch The property of a sound, especially a musical tone, that is determined by the frequency of the waves producing it; the highness or lowness of sound; the relative level, intensity, or extent of some quality or state.

tono Propiedad de un sonido, especialmente de un tono musical, que está determinada por la frecuencia de las ondas que lo producen; cualidad alta o baja de un sonido; nivel, intensidad o extensión relativos de alguna cualidad o estado.

policyholder The person who pays a premium to an insurance company (and in whose name the policy is written) in exchange for the insurance protection provided by a policy of insurance.

titular de la póliza Persona que paga una prima a una compañía aseguradora (y a cuyo nombre se contrata la póliza) a cambio de la cobertura que proporciona una póliza de seguro.

portfolio A set of pictures, drawings, documents, or photographs either bound in book form or loose in a folder.

portafolio Conjunto de ilustraciones, dibujos, documentos o fotografías, organizadas ya sea archivadas en forma de libro, o sueltas en una carpeta.

posting To transfer or carry from a book of original entry to a ledger; to enter figures in an accounting system.

asentar Transferir o traer desde un libro de entradas originales a un libro mayor; entrar cifras en un sistema de contabilidad.

postmortem Done, collected, or occurring after death.

postmortem Hecho, recogido o sucedido después de la muerte.

power of attorney A legal instrument authorizing a person to act as the attorney or agent of the grantor. The authority may be limited to the handling of specific procedures. The person authorized to act as the agent is known as the *attorney in fact*.

potestad legal Instrumento legal que autoriza a una persona a actuar como abogado o agente de la persona que le concede el poder. La autorización puede estar limitada al manejo de procedimientos específicos. La persona autorizada a actuar como agente se conoce como *abogado de hecho*.

precedence Superiority in rank, dignity, or importance; the condition of being, going, or coming ahead or in front of.

precedencia Superioridad en rango, dignidad o importancia; condición de estar, ir o venir primero o antes.

precedent A person or thing that serves as a model; something done or said that may serve as an example or rule to authorize or justify a subsequent act of the same kind.

precedente Persona o cosa que sirve como modelo; algo hecho o dicho anteriormente y que puede servir como ejemplo o norma para autorizar o justificar un acto subsiguiente del mismo tipo.

preexisting condition A physical condition of an insured person that existed before the issuance of the insurance policy.

afección preexistente Afección física de una persona asegurada que ya existía antes de la emisión de la póliza de seguro.

premium The consideration paid for a contract of insurance; the periodic (monthly, quarterly, or annual) payment of a specific sum of money to an insurance company that, in return, agrees to provide certain benefits.

prima Pago por un contrato de seguro; pago periódico (mensual, trimestral o anual) de una suma específica de dinero a una compañía aseguradora, la cual, a cambio, acepta proporcionar ciertos beneficios.

preponderance A superiority or excess in number or quantity; majority.

preponderancia Superioridad o mayor número o cantidad; mayoría.

preponderance of the evidence Evidence that is of greater weight or more convincing than the evidence offered in opposition to it; evidence that, as a whole, shows that the fact sought to be proven is more probable than not.

preponderancia de evidencia Evidencia que tiene mayor peso o que es más convincente que la evidencia con la que se confronta; evidencia que, en conjunto, muestra que el hecho que se pretende probar es más posible que imposible.

prerequisite Something that is necessary to achieve a result or to carry out a function.

requisito previo Algo que es necesario para obtener un resultado o para desempeñar una función.

pressboard A strong, highly glazed composition board resembling vulcanized fiber; heavy card stock.

cartón prensado Cartón de composición resistente y muy satinado que se parece a la fibra vulcanizada; cartulina de gran resistencia.

primary diagnosis The condition or chief complaint for which a patient is treated in outpatient (physician's office or clinic) medical care.
diagnóstico primario Afección o problema principal por el cual se trata a un paciente con atención médica externa (en un consultorio médico o una clínica).

principal A capital sum of money due as a debt or used as a fund, for which interest is either charged or paid.
principal Capital o suma de dinero que se debe como deuda o que se usa como fondo, por el cual se cargan o se cobran intereses.

principal diagnosis A condition, established after study, that is chiefly responsible for the *admission* of a patient to the hospital. It is used in coding inpatient hospital insurance claims.
diagnóstico principal Enfermedad o lesión que, tras su estudio, se determina que es la causa principal por la que un paciente *ingresa* en el hospital. Es usado en la codificación de reclamaciones de seguros de pacientes hospitalizados.

privately owned laboratories (POLs) Laboratories owned by a private individual or corporation, such as a free-standing laboratory or the lab inside a physician's office.
laboratorios privados (POLs) Laboratorios cuyo propietario es un individuo o una corporación privada, como el laboratorio dentro de un consultorio médico o un laboratorio independiente.

processing How an individual internalizes new information and makes it his or her own.
procesar Forma en la que un individuo interioriza y asimila la información nueva.

procrastination Intentionally putting off the doing of something that should be done.
procrastinación Dejar a un lado o retrasar, de manera intencional, algo que debe hacerse.

professional behaviors Those actions that identify the Medical Assistant as a member of a healthcare profession, including dependability, respectful patient care, initiative, positive attitude, and teamwork.
comportamientos profesionales Características que identifican al asistente médico como profesional de la atención sanitaria, incluyendo confiabilidad, trato respetuoso a los pacientes, iniciativa, actitud positiva y disposición para trabajar en equipo.

professional courtesy Reduction or absence of a fee to professional associates.
cortesía profesional Reducción o supresión de un cargo para los asociados profesionales.

professionalism Characterizing or conforming to the technical or ethical standards of a profession; exhibiting a courteous, conscientious, and generally businesslike manner in the workplace.
profesionalismo Actitud que se caracteriza por cumplir o actuar de acuerdo con los estándares técnicos y éticos de una profesión; dar muestras de cortesía, meticulosidad y, en general, mostrar un comportamiento adecuado en el lugar de trabajo.

proficiency Competency as a result of training or practice.
pericia Estado de competencia en algo, que se alcanza por medio de entrenamiento o práctica.

profit sharing Offer of part of the company's profits to employees or other designated individuals or groups.
participación en los beneficios Oferta de parte de los beneficios de la compañía a los empleados u otros individuos o grupos designados.

progress notes Notes entered in the patient chart to track the progress and condition of the patient.
notas del progreso Notas escritas en historial médico del paciente para seguir el progreso y estado del mismo.

proofread To read text and mark corrections.
corregir pruebas Leer un texto y marcar correcciones.

prosthesis The artificial replacement for a body part.
prótesis Pieza artificial para reemplazar una parte del cuerpo.

provider An individual or company that provides medical care and services to patients or the public.
proveedor Individuo o compañía que proporciona atenciones y servicios médicos pacientes o al público.

provisional diagnosis A temporary diagnosis made prior to receiving all test results.
diagnóstico provisional Diagnóstico temporal llevado a cabo antes de recibir todos los resultados de las pruebas.

proxemics The study of the nature, degree, and effect of the spatial separation individuals naturally maintain.
proxemia Estudio de la naturaleza, grado y efecto de la separación espacial que los individuos mantienen de forma natural.

prudent Marked by wisdom or judiciousness; shrewd in the management of practical affairs.
prudente Caracterizado por poseer sabiduría o sensatez; hábil en el manejo de los asuntos prácticos.

psychosocial Pertaining to a combination of psychological and social factors.
psicosocial Perteneciente o relativo a una combinación de factores psicológicos y sociales.

public domain The realm embracing property rights that belong to the community at large, are unprotected by copyright or patent, and are subject to appropriation by anyone.
dominio público Campo que abarca los derechos de propiedad que pertenecen a la comunidad en general, que no están protegidos por leyes de derechos de autor ni por patentes y están sujetos a apropiación por parte de cualquiera.

quackery The pretense of curing disease.
curanderismo Práctica del que finge curar enfermedades.

quality control An aggregate of activities designed to ensure adequate quality, especially in manufactured products or in the service industries.
control de calidad Conjunto de actividades destinadas a garantizar la calidad adecuada, en especial en productos manufacturados o en las industrias de servicios.

queries Requests for information from a database.
consultas Peticions de información de una base de datos.

ramifications Consequences produced by a cause or following from a set of conditions.
ramificaciones Consecuencias producidas por una causa o que siguen a una serie de estados.

rapport A relationship of harmony and accord between the patient and the health care professional.
concordia Relación de armonía y acuerdo entre el paciente y el profesional de la atención sanitaria.

RBRVS (resource-based relative value system) A fee schedule designed to provide national uniform payment of Medicare benefits after being adjusted to reflect the differences in practice costs across geographic areas.
RBRVS (sistema de valor relativo basado en recursos) Escala de cargos diseñada para proporcionar un pago de beneficios de Medicare uniforme a nivel nacional después de haber sido ajustado para reflejar las diferencias en los costos prácticos a través de áreas geográficas.

ream A quantity of paper consisting of 20 quires or variously 480, 500, or 516 sheets.
resma Una cantidad de papel que consiste de 20 manos o que varía entre 480, 500 o 516 hojas.

reasonable doubt Doubt based on reason and arising from evidence or lack of evidence; not doubt that is imagined or conjured up, but doubt that would cause reasonable persons to hesitate before acting in a manner important to themselves.
duda razonable Duda basada en la razón o que surge de evidencia o falta de evidencia; no es una duda imaginaria ni inventada, sino una duda que puede hacer que una persona razonable vacile antes de dar un paso importante.

receipts Amounts paid on patient accounts.
recibos Sumas pagadas en las cuentas de los pacientes.

recipient The receiver of some thing or item.
receptor El que recibe un artículo u objeto.

rectify To correct by removing errors.
rectificar Corregir eliminando errores.

referral (reference) laboratory A private or hospital-based laboratory that performs a wide variety of tests, many of them specialized. Physicians often send specimens collected in the office to referral laboratories for testing.
laboratorio de referencia Laboratorio privado o de un hospital que realiza una amplia gama de análisis, muchos de ellos especializados. Con frecuencia los médicos envían especímenes recogidos en la consulta a estos laboratorios para ser analizados.

reflection The process of considering new information and internalizing it to create new ways of examining information.
reflexión Proceso de estudiar información nueva e interiorizarla para crear formas nuevas de examinar información.

registered dietitian (RD) A professionally certified person with a bachelor's degree in food and nutrition who is concerned with the maintenance and promotion of health and the treatment of diseases through proper diet.
dietista registrado (RD) Profesional certificado persona con titulación universitaria en alimentos y nutrición y que se preocupa del mantenimiento y la promoción de la salud y el tratamiento de las enfermedades a través de la dieta adecuado.

relevant Having significant and demonstrable bearing on the matter at hand.
pertinente Que tiene una relación importante y demostrable con el asunto que se está tratando.

reparations The act of making amends, offering atonement, or giving satisfaction for a wrong or injury.
reparaciones Acción de enmendar u ofrecer compensaciones por un error o un daño.

reprimands Criticisms for a fault; a severe or formal reproof.
reprimendas Críticas por una falta; reprobación severa o formal.

reproach An expression of rebuke or disapproval; a cause or occasion of blame, discredit, or disgrace.
reproche Expresión de crítica o desaprobación; causa o motivo de culpa, descrédito u oprobio.

requisites Things considered essential or necessary.
requisitos Cosas que se consideran esenciales o necesarias.

retention schedule A method or plan for retaining or keeping track of medical records and their movement from active to inactive to closed filing.
plan de retención Método o plan para retener o guardar expedientes médicos, y el paso de los mismos del estado de expediente activo a pasivo y a cerrado.

retention Keeping something in possession or use; to keeping someone's pay or service.
retención El hecho de mantener en posesión o en uso; mantener a alguien a su servicio o como empleado.

retribution The giving or receiving of reward or punishment; something given or exacted in recompense.
retribución Acto de dar o recibir una recompensa o castigo; algo que se da o se cobra como recompensa.

rider A special provision or group of provisions added to an insurance policy to expand or limit the benefits otherwise payable. It may increase or decrease benefits, waive a condition or coverage, or in any other way amend the original contract.
cláusula adicional Provisión o conjunto de provisiones especiales añadidas a una póliza de seguro para ampliar o limitar los beneficios que de otro modo se pueden pagar. Puede aumentar o disminuir beneficios, anular una condición o cobertura o puede enmendar el contrato original de otra manera.

robotics Technology dealing with the design, construction, and operation of robots in automation.
robótica Tecnología de la automatización que se ocupa del diseño, construcción y operación de robots.

router A device used to connect any number of LANs which communicate with other routers and determine the best route between any two hosts.
direccionador Dispositivo usado para conectar cualquier cantidad de LAN que se comunican con otros direccionadores para determinar la mejor ruta entre dos computadoras conectadas a una red.

salutation Word or gestures expressing greeting, good will, or courtesy.
saludo Expresión de saludo, buenos deseos o cortesía por medio de palabras o gestos.

sarcasm A sharp and often satirical response or ironic utterance designed to cut or give pain.
sarcasmo Respuesta aguda y frecuentemente satírica o declaración irónica destinada a burlarse o a lastimar.

scanner A device that reads text or illustrations on a printed page and translates the information into a form that the computer can understand.
escáner Dispositivo que lee texto o ilustraciones de una página impresa y traduce esa información a un formato comprensible para la computadora.

screen Something that shields, protects, or hides; to select or eliminate products or applicants by comparing them to a set of desired criteria.
pantalla Algo que actúa como escudo, que protege u oculta para permitir un proceso de selección.

search engines Computer programs that search documents for keywords and return a list of documents containing those words.
buscadores Programas de computadoras que buscan documentos a partir de palabras clave y proporcionan una lista de los documentos que contienen esas palabras.

"see also" An instruction to the coder to look elsewhere if the main term or subterm(s) for an entry are not sufficient for coding the information. If a code number follows, "see also" is enclosed in parentheses; there is no code number, "see also" is preceded by a dash.
"ver también" Instrucción que se le da a la persona encargada de la codificación para que consulte en algún otro lugar si el término o subtérminos principales para una entrada no son suficientes para codificar la información. Si "ver también" va seguido por un número de código, dicho código va entre paréntesis; si no hay número de código, "ver también" va precedido por un guión.

"see category" An instruction to the coder to refer to a specific category (three-digit code); it must always be followed.
"ver categoría" Instrucción que se le da a la persona encargada de la codificación para que consulte una categoría específica (código de tres dígitos); Siempre debe seguirse.

"see" An instruction to the coder to look in another place. This instruction must always be followed and is found in the Alphabetic Index, volumes 2 and 3.
"ver" Instrucción que se le da a la persona encargada de la codificación para que consulte en otro lugar. Siempre debe seguirse esta instrucción; la expresión se encuentra en el Índice alfabético, tomos 2 y 3.

self-insured plans Insurance plans funded by organizations having a big enough employee base that they can afford to fund their own insurance program.
planes de autoaseguración Planes de seguros implementados por organizaciones con un número de empleados lo suficientemente grande como para permitirles financiar su propio programa de seguros.

sequentially Happening in relation to or by arrangement in a sequence.
secuencial Aquello que ocurre relativo a una secuencia o que es ordenado en secuencia.

service benefit plan A plan that provides benefits in the form of certain surgical and medical services rendered, rather than in cash. A service benefit plan is not restricted to a fee schedule.
plan de beneficios de servicio Plan que proporciona beneficios en forma de ciertos servicios médico-quirúrgicos en vez de con dinero en metálico. Un plan de servicio de beneficio no está restringido por una escala de cargos.

shingling A method of filing whereby each new report is laid on top of the next older report, resembling the shingles of a roof.
laminado Método de archivo en el cual cada informe nuevo se coloca encima del informe anterior, del mismo modo que se colocan las tejas en un techo.

socioeconomic Relating to a combination of social and economic factors.
socioeconómico Perteneciente o relativo a una combinación de factores sociales y económicos.

sociological Oriented or directed toward social needs and problems.
sociologico Que se orienta o dirige hacia las necesidades y problemas sociales.

sound card A device that allows a computer to output sound through speakers that are connected to the main circuitry board (motherboard).
tarjeta de sonido Dispositivo que le permite a una computadora emitir sonido a través de altavoces conectados a la tarjeta principal del circuito.

staff privileges Authorization for a healthcare professional to practice within a specific facility.
privilegios del personal Autorización para un profesional de atención sanitaria, para ejercer la práctica dentro de unas instalaciones específicas.

standards Items or indicators used to measure quality or compliance with a statutory or accrediting body's policies and regulations.
estándares Artículos o indicadores usados para medir la calidad o cumplimiento de las pólizas

y regulaciones de un cuerpo normativo o acreditativo.

stat Medical abbreviation for immediately or at this moment; an order found on a laboratory requisition indicating that the test must be done immediately (from the Latin word *statin*, meaning "at once"); immediately.
stat Abreviatura usada en medicina que significa inmediatamente o ahora mismo. Orden encontrada en un pedido de laboratorio que indica que el análisis debe llevarse a cabo inmediatamente (de la palabra latina *statin,* que significa "ahora"); inmediatamente.

stationers Sellers of writing paper.
dependientes de papelería Vendedores de artículos de papelería.

statute A law enacted by the legislative branch of a government.
estatuto Ley sancionada por la rama legislativa de un gobierno.

stereotype Something conforming to a fixed or general pattern; a standardized mental picture that is held in common by many and represents an oversimplified opinion, prejudiced attitude, or uncritical judgment.
estereotipo Algo que se ajusta a un patrón fijado o general; imagen mental estandarizada que tienen en común muchas personas y que representa opiniones simplificadas, actitudes con prejuicios o razonamientos carentes de sentido crítico.

stipulate To specify as a condition or requirement of an agreement or offer; to make an agreement or covenant to do or forbear something.
estipular Especificar como condición o requisito de un acuerdo u oferta; establecer un acuerdo o prometer hacer, o dejar de hacer, algo.

stock option Offer of stocks for purchase to a certain individual or to certain groups, such as employees of a for-profit hospital.
opción sobre acciones Oferta de venta de acciones que se le hace a un ciertos individuos o grupos, como a los empleados de un hospital.

stressors Stimuli that cause stress.
estresantes Dícese de los estímulos que causan estrés.

subjective information Information gained by questioning the patient or taking it from a form.
información subjetiva Información obtenida haciendo preguntas al paciente o tomándola de un formulario.

subluxations Slight misalignments of the vertebrae, or a partial dislocation.
subluxaciones Alineamientos ligeramente defectuosos o dislocaciones parciales de las vértebras.

subordinate Submissive to or controlled by authority; placed in or occupying a lower class, rank, or position.
subordinado Que está sometido a una autoridad o controlado por ella; que ostenta un cargo u ocupa una clase, rango o puesto inferior.

subpoena A writ or document commanding a person to appear in court, under penalty for failure to appear.
subpoena Documento escrito ordenando a una persona comparecer en el juzgado bajo penalidad en caso de no comparecencia.

substance number A number based on the weight of a ream of paper containing 500 sheets.
número de sustancia Número basado en el peso de una resma de papel de 500 hojas.

subtle Difficult to understand or perceive; having or marked by keen insight and the ability to penetrate deeply and thoroughly.
sutil Difícil de comprender o percibir; que tiene perspicacia y la capacidad de penetrar a fondo y en toda su extensión en un asunto.

succinct Marked by compact, precise expression without wasted words.
sucinto Caracterizado por una expresión precisa y concisa sin palabras inútiles.

superfluous Exceeding what is sufficient or necessary.
superfluos Que exceden aquello que es suficiente o necesario.

surrogate A substitute; put in place of another.
subrogado Sustituto; puesto en lugar de otro.

switch In networks, a device that filters information between LAN segments, decreases overall network traffic, and increases speed and bandwidth usage efficiency.
conmutador En las redes de comunicación, dispositivo que filtra información entre segmentos de LAN y disminuye el tráfico global de la red, aumentando la velocidad y la eficacia en el uso del ancho de banda.

synopsis A condensed statement or outline.
sinopsis Declaración resumida; resumen.

tactful Having a keen sense of what to do or say in order to maintain good relations with others or avoid offense.
tacto Tener un sentido de lo que se debe hacer o decir para mantener buenas relaciones con los demás y evitar ofenderlos.

targeted to Directed or used toward a target; directed toward a specific desire or position.
dirigido a Dirigido a un fin o meta específico, usado hacia un fin; dirigido hacia un deseo o un puesto específico.

TCP/IP Abbreviation for Transmission Control Protocol/Internet Protocol; a suite of communications protocols used to connect users or hosts to the Internet.
TCP/IP Abreviatura de protocolo de control de transmisión/protocolo Internet; conjunto de protocolos de comunicación que se usa para conectar usuarios o computadoras a Internet.

tedious Tiresome because of length or dullness.
tedioso Que cansa porque es demasiado largo o aburrido.

telecommunications The science and technology of communication by transmission of information from one location to another via telephone, television, telegraph, or satellite.
telecomunicaciones Ciencia y tecnología de la comunicación basada en la transmisión de información de un lugar a otro por teléfono, televisión, telégrafo o satélite.

telemedicine The use of telecommunications in the practice of medicine, allowing great distances between healthcare professionals, colleagues, patients, and students.
telemedicina Uso de las telecomunicaciones en la práctica médica, permitiendo la comunicación entre profesionales de atención sanitaria, colegas, pacientes y estudiantes que se hallan a grandes distancias.

teleradiology The use of telecommunications devices to enhance and improve the results of radiological procedures.
telerradiología Uso de dispositivos de telecomunicación para mejorar y perfeccionar los resultados de procedimientos radiológicos.

testimony A solemn declaration usually made orally by a witness under oath in response to interrogation by a lawyer or authorized public official.
testimonio Declaración solemne, por lo general oral, hecha por un testigo bajo juramento como respuesta a una pregunta (o preguntas) de un abogado o un funcionario público autorizado.

thanatology The description or study of the phenomena of death and of psychological methods of coping with death.
tanatología Descripción o estudio del fenómeno de la muerte y de los métodos psicológicos para hacerle frente.

third-party payer An entity (usually an insurance company) that makes a payment on an obligation or debt but is not a party to the contract that created the debt.
pagador mediador Entidad (por lo general una compañía aseguradora) que hace un pago de una obligación o deuda pero que no es parte del contrato que ha creado dicha deuda.

third-party payer Someone other than the patient, spouse, or parent who is responsible for paying all or part of the patient's medical costs.
pagador mediador Alguien ajeno al paciente, cónyuge, padre o madre que es responsable del pago de todo o parte de los gastos médicos del paciente o de parte de ellos.

tickler file A chronological file used as a reminder that something must be taken care of on a certain date.
archivo cronológico Archivo que se usa para recordar que algo que debe llevarse a cabo en una fecha determinada.

transaction An exchange or transfer of goods, services, or funds.
transacción Intercambio o transferencia de bienes, servicios o fondos.

transcription A written copy made either in longhand or by machine.
transcripción Copia escrita de algo, hecha a mano, o con la ayuda de una máquina.

treatises Systematic expositions or arguments in writing, including methodical discussion of the facts and principles involved and the conclusions reached.
tratados Exposiciones sistemáticas o argumentos escritos que incluyen una descripción metódica de los hechos y principios involucrados y las conclusiones a las que se ha llegado.

triage Responding to requests for immediate care and treatment after evaluating the urgency of the need and prioritizing the treatment; the sorting and allocation of treatment to patients according to a system of priorities designed to maximize the number of survivors and treat the sickest patients first.
criterio de selección Responder a peticiones de atención y tratamiento inmediato tras evaluar la urgencia de la necesidad y establecer prioridades de tratamiento. Clasificación y asignación de tratamiento a pacientes según un sistema de prioridades destinado a maximizar el número de sobrevivientes y tratar primero a los pacientes más enfermos.

Uniform Commercial Code A unified set of rules covering many business transactions; often referred to simply as the UCC, it has been adopted in all 50 states, the District of Columbia, and most U.S. territories.
Código de Comercio Uniforme (UCC) Conjunto de normas unificadas que cubren muchas transacciones comerciales; se conoce simplemente como UCC y ha sido adoptado en los 50 estados, el Distrito de Columbia y la mayoría de los territorios estadounidenses.

unique identifiers A method of anonymous HIV testing in which a code is used, instead of names, to protect the confidentiality of the patient.
identificadores únicos Método de prueba de VIH (HIV) anónimo en el cual se usa un código en lugar de nombres, para proteger la confidencialidad del paciente.

universal claim form The form developed by the Health Care Financing Administration (HCFA, now known as the Centers for Medicare and Medicaid Services, or CMS) and approved by the AMA for use in submitting all government sponsored claims.
formulario de reclamación universal Formulario desarrollado por la Administración financiera de la atención sanitaria (HCFA, ahora conocida como Centros de servicios de Medicare y Medicaid, o CMS) y aprobado por AMA para usarse al someter todas las reclamaciones subvencionadas por el gobierno.

URL Abbreviation for Uniform Resource Locator; the global address of documents or information on the Internet. The URL provides the IP address and the domain name for the web page, such as *microsoft.com."*
URL Abreviatura de localizador universal de recursos; la dirección a nivel mundial, de documentos o de información en Internet. El URL proporciona la dirección IP y el nombre del dominio de una página web, como por ejemplo: *microsoft.com."*

"use additional code" This term appears only in volume 1 in those subdivisions where the user should add further information by means of an additional code to give a more complete picture of the diagnosis. In some cases you will find "if desired" following the term. For the purpose of coding in military medical treatment facilities, the "if desired" phrase will not be used. Therefore when the term "use additional code ... if desired" appears, you will disregard "if desired" and assign the appropriate additional code.
"usar código adicional" Esta expresión aparece sólo en el tomo 1, en aquellas subdivisiones en las que el usuario debe añadir más información por medio de un código adicional para proporcionar un cuadro más completo del diagnóstico. En algunos casos, se verá "si se desea" tras el término. En la codificación en establecimientos militares de tratamiento médico, no se usará la expresión "si se desea". Por lo tanto, cuando aparezca el término "usar código adicional ... si se desea", no se tendrá en cuenta "si se desea" y se asignará el código adicional correspondiente.

utilization review The review of individual cases by a committee to make sure that services are medically necessary and to study how providers use medical care resources.
revisión de utilización Revisión de casos individuales por un comité, para asegurarse de

que los servicios son médicamente necesarios y estudiar cómo los proveedores usan los recursos de cuidados de salud.

veracity Devotion to or conformity with the truth.
veracidad Compromiso o conformidad con la verdad.

verdict The finding or decision of a jury on a matter submitted to it in trial.
veredicto Conclusión o decisión de un jurado en un asunto sometido a juicio.

versatile Embracing a variety of subjects, fields or skills; having a wide range of abilities.
versátil Que abarca diferentes sujetos, campos o destrezas; que tiene una amplia gama de destrezas.

vested Granted or endowed with a particular authority, right, or property; having a special interest in something.
conferirido Concedido o dotado con una autoridad, derecho o propiedad particular; que tiene un interés especial en algo.

virtual reality An artificial environment, experienced by a computer user often using special gloves, earphones, and goggles to enhance the experience, that feels as if it were a real environment.
realidad virtual Entorno artificial que experimenta el usuario de una computadora, muchas veces usando guantes especiales, audífonos y lentes para mejorar la experiencia, y que parece ser un ambiente real.

vocation The work in which a person is regularly employed.
profesión Trabajo en el que una persona está empleada regularmente.

volatile Referring to a flammable substance's capacity to vaporize at a low temperature. Easily aroused; tending to erupt in violence.
volátil Referente a la capacidad de una sustancia flamable para evaporarse a baja temperatura. Que reacciona con facilidad y tiene tendencia a entrar en erupción de forma violenta.

watermark A mark in paper resulting from differences in thickness usually produced by pressure of a projecting design in the mold or on a processing roll, and visible when the paper is held up to the light.
filigrana Marca en un papel que resulta de diferencias de espesor, por lo general se produce presionando un diseño en relieve en el molde o en un rodillo de procesamiento, y es visible por transparencia.

"with" In the context of ICD-9-CM, the terms "with," "with mention of," or "associated with" in a title dictates that both parts of the title must be present in the statement of the diagnosis in order to assign the particular code.
"con" En el contexto de la ICD-9-CM, las expresiones "con", "con mención de" y "asociado con" en un título exigen que ambas partes del título estén presentes en la descripción del orden de diagnóstico para asignar el código específico.

workers' compensation Insurance against liability imposed on certain employers to pay benefits and furnish care to employees injured, and to pay benefits to dependents of employees killed, in the course of or arising out of their employment.
compensación laboral Seguro contra la responsabilidad impuesta a ciertos patronos para pagar beneficios y proporcionar atenciones a los trabajadores lesionados, y pagar beneficios a las personas que dependan de trabajadores que mueran en el trabajo o a causa de él.

Zip drive A small and portable disk drive that is primarily used for backing up information and archiving computer files; a 100 megabyte zip disk will hold the equivalent of about 70 floppy disks.
Unidad zip Unidad de un disco pequeño y portátil que se usa principalmente para hacer copias de seguridad de información y para guardar archivos electrónicos. Un disco zip de 100 megabytes tiene una capacidad equivalente a la de unos 70 disquetes.

Credits

Page 299 constitutes an extension of the copyright page. The illustrations that appear on the pages listed below are from the following sources.

From Davis N, Lacour M: *Introduction to health information technology,* Philadelphia, 2002, WB Saunders.
Pages 51, 56, 76-81, 120-122, 131-132

From Hunt SA, Zonderman JH: *Saunders fundamentals of medical assisting: student mastery manual,* Philadelphia, 2002, WB Saunders.
Pages 58-59, 67, 70, 73, 85-89, 100, 104, 113-116, 118, 136-137, 139

From Young T, Kennedy D: *Kinn's the medical assistant: an applied learning approach,* 9th ed., Philadelphia, 2003, Elsevier Science (USA).
Pages 29, 94, 97-98, 101-103